the
no-nonsense
meditation book

Praise for *The No-Nonsense Meditation Book*

'Clear, lively, rigorous and authentic... The book we have been waiting for.'
Ilios Kotsou, PhD, Chair in Mindfulness, Grenoble School of Management

'Steven Laureys' book opens up exciting perspectives.'
Matthieu Ricard, PhD, Buddhist monk & translator of the Dalai Lama

'Not reading this is self-defeating.'
Paul Witteman, Dutch journalist and TV presenter

'Dr Laureys provides an unusually cogent and compelling description of different forms of meditation and why we should care about them. The book is both a tutorial and a guide, and helps the reader understand large bodies of scientific work — and their implications for everyday life. This book gives new meaning to the idea of "mental exercise", and I recommend it to all who seek to have more focused and directed behaviour and a deeper understanding of their place in the world.'
Stephen M. Kosslyn, PhD, President Emeritus, Harvard University Foundry College

'I have known for some time that I should be meditating, but have always found some reason not to. This brilliant book has banished all those reasons. Laureys really does cut out all the nonsense and provides the clearest-yet description of meditation and its benefits. He will change (and save) lives.'
Trevor Harley, FBPsS, Emeritus Professor of Psychology,
University of Dundee, Scotland

'By weaving the neuroscience of consciousness with the contemplative roots of compassion with easy-to-follow meditation instructions, into a personal story, this book pulls you in and might just change your life. The clarity and simplicity of Dr Laureys' voice makes it feel like he is in the room with you and his humor and scepticism, about nearly everything, makes this book an easy and delightful read.'
Nancy E. Oriol, MD, Harvard Medical School, Boston

'In Steven Laureys' beautiful and timely book, both hard-core scientists and contemplative practitioners will find inspiration and guidance ... *The No-Nonsense Meditation Book* is a wonderful amalgamation of scientific rigor with touching, compassionate, and humble curiosity.'
Diego Hangartner, Co-Founder of Mind and Life Europe

'This book, describing one Belgian neurologist's journey from sceptic to advocate, provides an excellent overview of our current neuroscientific understanding of meditation, and its potential role in health and disease.'
Jerome Engel, MD, PhD, Professor of Neurology, UCLA, Los Angeles

Steven Laureys MD

the
no-nonsense
meditation book

A scientist's guide
to the power of
meditation

GREEN TREE
LONDON · OXFORD · NEW YORK · NEW DELHI · SYDNEY

GREEN TREE
Bloomsbury Publishing Plc
50 Bedford Square, London, WC1B 3DP, UK
29 Earlsfort Terrace, Dublin 2, Ireland

BLOOMSBURY, GREEN TREE and the Green Tree logo are trademarks
of Bloomsbury Publishing Plc

First published in 2019 in Belgium as *Het no-nonsense meditatieboek*
by Borgerhoff & Lamberigts

First published in Great Britain 2021

Translated by Henriette Korthals Altes

A catalogue record for this book is available from the British Library

Library of Congress Cataloguing-in-Publication data has been applied for

ISBN: HB: 978-1-4729-8049-6; eBook: 978-1-4729-8050-2;
ePdf: 978-1-4729-8047-2

4 6 8 10 9 7 5 3

Typeset in Minion Pro by Deanta Global Publishing Services, Chennai, India
Printed and bound in Great Britain by CPI Group (UK) Ltd, Croydon, CR0 4YY

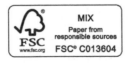

To find out more about our authors and books visit www.bloomsbury.com
and sign up for our newsletters

*To all my patients, colleagues, health workers, students, contemplative monks,
who taught me to appreciate the power of meditation.
To my admirable children, Clara, Hugo, Matias, Louis, Margot, who have all
have been a source of inspiration, ethics and mindfulness in action.
To my wife Vanessa, the sunshine of my life.*

Contents

~

8

Foreword

Our mind can be both our best friend and worst enemy. There are times when the outside world feels like it's in a state of turmoil, because you are in a state of turmoil inside. Rehashing the past, anticipating possible troubles, and failing to manage our deeply ingrained thought patterns can be so difficult that it destroys our enthusiasm for life. In order to heal inner suffering, training your mind to meditate can be invaluable.

Steven Laureys' book offers plenty of inspiration, with both its clear presentation and its rigorous scientific explanations. It encourages us all not to underestimate the potential for our brain to transform, to fully realise this potential and thus become better human beings, for our own benefit and for the greater good of those around us. As the story of how he overcame the challenges that life threw at him unfolds, Steven allows us to discover not only the meditation techniques that have helped him in his own personal journey, but also the scientific investigations he undertook as he met with experienced meditators.

It was a great joy to become Steven's friend and collaborate with him on cutting-edge scientific studies that looked at the interface between meditation and the workings of the mind. My own contribution was only a humble one, but I was fascinated by the new experimental techniques that allowed him to measure levels of 'contentment' and 'presence', of consciousness, not only in the injured brain, which is what Steven specialises in, but also in states of wakefulness and states induced by the person who meditates, ranging from opaque sleepiness to extreme lucidity.

In his book Steven often refers to my modest participation in his experiments, but it is important to know that the encouraging findings of his research do not relate to individuals who possess extraordinary capacities, but to skills that each of us can learn over time.

Other studies, particularly those led by the neuroscientists Richard David-son and Antoine Lutz, focusing both on Tibetan monks, and men and women from diverse social backgrounds, have found that all those who have followed the same meditative practices over a period of years show similar changes in the working and structure of their brains. Therefore, it is practice, and not the individual subject, that determines the scope of the experiment's results.

In these types of studies, the meditator is primarily a docile guinea pig, as he is tested for up to eight hours a day! But he also actively collaborates in so far as he is the only one who can account for what he experiences on a personal level when he enters into various meditative states, ranging from 'open presence' and 'focused attention' to 'unconditional loving kindness'. On the one hand, researchers mainly take a third-person approach – they study the states of the brain using various techniques – and a second-per-son approach – they use a questionnaire about what participants in the experiment have experienced. Yet only the meditator themselves is in a position to offer true interpretations of the scientific data from their first-person perspective.

In what ways can we train the mind to function constructively to replace obsession with contentment, restlessness with peacefulness, and hatred with compassion? About 20 years ago, a quasi-dogmatic position prevai-led, which held that the brain contained all its neurons at birth and that its structure did not vary much according to experience. Nowadays, 'neu-roplasticity' is the notion that holds currency, a term that accounts for the fact that the brain constantly evolves according to our experiences, and produces new neurons and connections throughout our lives. Indeed, the brain can be thoroughly modified thanks to specific training, such as learning to play a musical instrument or taking up a new form of exercise, as well as practising meditation. This means that attention, compassion and even happiness can be cultivated, and are 'know-how' that can be acquired.

Acquiring know-how requires training. Nobody can expect to play the piano fluently or tennis at a certain level without lengthy training. Like-wise, if you dedicate a certain time every day to the cultivation of compas-sion or any other positive quality, you can easily see how you can obtain results similar to those reached with a physical workout. When it comes to Buddhism, to meditate means to 'get used to' or to 'cultivate'; it means to familiarise oneself with a new mode of being, of managing your thoughts and perceiving the world. In order to do so you must practise assiduously for months and years.

Today neuroscience allows us to evaluate these methods and verify their impact on the brain and the body. Numerous studies have shown that it is not necessary to be highly trained in meditation in order to enjoy its benefits, and that 20 minutes of daily practice can contribute significantly to lowering anxiety and stress levels, while strengthening immunity and emotional balance. The Silver Santé European programme, for instance, which studies the effect of meditation on ageing, has yielded very promising results.[1]

The Dalai Lama considers Buddhism to be first and foremost a science of the mind. This should not come as a surprise, since Buddhist texts insist on the fact that all spiritual practices, be they mental, physical or verbal, have the objective, directly or indirectly, of transforming the mind. As Yongey Mingyur Rinpoche, another Buddhist master who collaborates with eminent scientists, has explained, 'One of the main difficulties met when examining one's mind is the deep-seated, often unconscious, belief that one is what one is and that changing oneself is impossible. I have experienced this feeling of unhelpful pessimism as a child and I have often observed it in others as I have travelled around the world. Although we are not conscious of it, the idea that our mind cannot change precludes all attempts at change.'[2]

The constant concern shown by the 14th Dalai Lama for his human brothers and sisters, and his long-lasting interest in scientific discoveries, led to the creation of the Mind & Life Institute by the late cognitive scientist Francisco Varela and Adam Engle. This institute gathers around the Dalai Lama a group of world-class scientists and since 1985 it has organised a series of exciting conferences, in which I myself regularly take part.

In November 2005, when the Dalai Lama was invited to give the opening plenary at the Society for Neuroscience's annual meeting, which was attended by at least 37,000 scientists, he highlighted how Buddhism is essentially pragmatic and experimental, because it aims to dispel suffering through a better knowledge of the workings of the mind. He also asserted that if ancient Buddhist texts contradicted today's scientific findings, as is the case in the domain of cosmology, for instance, then their contents should be considered obsolete. 'On the other hand,' he added, 'Buddhism can share with modern science its knowledge of more than 2000 years of training the brain.'

For his part, Stephen Kosslyn, former director of the Psychology Department at Harvard University, explained at a Mind & Life meeting organised at MIT, in Cambridge, Massachusetts, that, 'We need to be humble before the mass of empirical data provided by contemplative Buddhists.' In the same spirit, Steven Laureys' book opens up exciting fresh perspectives in the new field of contemplative neuroscience research.[3]

Matthieu Ricard, Buddhist monk and scientist

~

Introduction

'You don't have to control your thoughts. You just have to stop letting them control you.'

DAN MILLMAN, trampoline world champion and author

One day, about a century ago, an old Japanese Zen master received a visit from a university professor who wanted to practise Zen meditation. The wise man started by giving him a cup of tea. He filled the cup to the brim, but against all expectations, he did not stop pouring. Surprised, the professor first watched his cup brimming over and then could not help saying to his host: 'Sir, the tea is spilling over, you need to stop.' The old man looked the professor in the eye and told him softly: 'You see, your brain is a bit like this cup. It brims over with thoughts, worries and opinions. Until you empty it, I won't be able to teach you anything about Zen meditation.'

I am a medical doctor and a man of science. As such, I would like to start by clarifying why writing this book and telling the stories within it means so much to me; why I want to explain how I use meditation in my neurology clinic at the hospital; and why I care so much about presenting the scientific findings of my lab and other research centres around the world. My professional journey is a rather traditional one. When I studied medicine, I learned a lot about the human body and the brain, about illnesses and the treatments to cure or face them. Later on, my research team and I focused on human states of consciousness, and now the damaged or unconscious brain has become my specialism. Thanks to the work and studies I carry out in our lab and clinical research centre at Liège, I have progressively come up with answers to the questions I had when I was a teenager. What is the purpose of our life on earth? Why do we think? How can we become better human beings? What is the meaning of life? I have had the opportunity to further my knowledge about human states of consciousness, about anaesthesia and about hypnosis, a technique we have studied thoroughly at the University Hospital of Liège. Each time I have learned a little more about the human brain; about our states of mind and our thought processes; about the reasons why our brain is constantly in turmoil and constantly evolving; and about what happens when something stimulates it.

Far be it from me to boast about what I know and what I have done. Like you, I loathe egocentric attitudes, personality cults or the adoration of an individual. What I am trying to convey by summarising my professional journey is that none of the knowledge I had acquired when I studied medicine or as a man of science helped me when, on 17 August 2012, my whole world suddenly collapsed. It was a real shock. I found myself alone with three children aged seven, 11 and 13. Until that day, I had always worked long, irregular hours in order to spend my free time with my family. All of a sudden, I was completely lost emotionally. I was a father, but I had also been a spouse, and my unexpected divorce left me profoundly shaken as a man. In spite of all my studies and all the books I had read, no therapy seemed able to relieve my suffering. No pills, ointment or operation would solve the problem.

I have nothing to hide and I don't have any issues about admitting that I went through really tough times during the first year after the breakup. I was unable to lead a healthy life. I threw myself into cigarettes and alcohol to overcome stress. I no longer took time off for myself, for my body or my mind. I was all over the place, trying to reconcile my career and family life. I even took anti-depressants and sleeping pills. After a rough patch lasting several months, I hit rock bottom and understood I could not continue in this way. I wanted to have my life back and to be inspiring for my kids. When this happens to you, the moment inevitably comes when you have to think of yourself. And in order to reconnect with myself I saw several therapists and psychiatrists.

I delved into books that could potentially help me face up to my issues. I started training for the marathon and found an outlet in yoga, which I took up on the advice of wise friends. Both the books I read and the yoga I practised each week led me to take a real interest in meditation. Of course, I had heard of it before, but like many of my colleagues in the scientific community, I was rather sceptical about it. Indeed, a few years before, when a journalist had asked me what I thought about mindfulness, which is one of the key pillars of meditation, I brushed the question aside. It was just hype, a fad encouraged by magazines and the Internet. But the more I read about it, the less clear-cut my position became.

The yoga meditation classes and the attitude of my teacher also raised my curiosity. I had already tried out many sports, but never reached a competitive level because of my non-conformist spirit. For instance, when my tennis teacher corrected my technique, I would, on purpose, hold my racquet a bit higher or move it too much to the right or to the left. The strictness of these training sessions did not fit either my rebel nature or my stubborn character. Yoga, in contrast, drew me in. The teacher didn't pay attention to the exact position of my left foot or whether I was able to reach my knees with my nose. What mattered during these yoga and breathing meditation classes were how I felt and my own progression; the things I learnt about myself, about my body and my state of mind in the moment.

This state of mind caught my interest as a neurologist. The little spare time I had, or that I took, I dedicated to reading books about philosophy, meditation, Christian contemplative practices and the Buddhist vision of life. As I grew into the topic, I naturally started living a more aware life. I didn't feel the need to complain about my past any longer or worry about the future. I just wanted to enjoy and live in the moment with my fabulous children. That's when I understood that mindfulness was not just a fad, as I had told the journalist a few years before, but instead a real added value to many aspects of our daily life, such as making the most of a good meal, thinking about how to organise your time or, when on holiday, not simply charging around from one tourist highlight to another, but taking the time to stop and admire the beauty of the moment.

From then on meditation started to play an important role in my daily routine, and also in my professional life. At the lab at the University of Liège, it was only a small step from our research on states of consciousness during hypnosis to research on states of mind during meditation. My scientific curiosity was really stimulated when I first met Matthieu Ricard, a doctor in molecular biology, Buddhist monk and French interpreter for the 14th Dalai Lama. It was a chance encounter that allowed me to exchange ideas with a man who was quite a character and whose books on Oriental philosophy, meditation and Buddhism I had read. We first met at a TEDx conference in Paris on 28 November 2013. These conferences gather together speakers who come to discuss topics and ideas 'worth spreading' linked to science, technology, business, sociology and creativity. Both of us were invited to this Paris edition. Even if I couldn't listen to all Matthieu had to say about the importance of altruism in the 21st century, his presence caught my attention. To my great joy, we nevertheless had some time to talk after the conference. For reasons that still remain obscure to me today, we immediately connected, although I can only vaguely remember the topic of our conversation. However, I do remember very clearly that he replied, 'Yes, with pleasure,' when I invited him to my lab in Liège, so that my research team could study his brain and the effects of the meditation that he had been practising for so many years.

It was not the first time he had participated in such studies. Ever since he decided to dedicate his life to Buddhism, and thus to meditation, several scientists have subjected him to tests aimed at showing the effects of meditative practices on the development and workings of the brain, and I wanted to continue to explore this data, with Matthieu as the perfect guinea pig.

Alongside our research collaboration on meditation, Matthieu also invited me to take part in a Mind & Life retreat. Mind & Life was created in 1987 in the United States with the aim of establishing a dialogue between modern neuroscience and the meditative traditions. In other words, it is an institute that facilitates a bridge between contemplative science, which has explored the workings of the mind for centuries, and contemporary science. The timing couldn't have been better! Vanessa, my new partner, a Canadian psychologist whom I married three years later, joined me in August 2014 for the first Mind & Life Europe summer school, which took place in a Christian nunnery in the idyllic setting of the Chiemsee islands in Germany. Matthieu came to present a paper, but also to teach meditation. It was my first true experience of formal meditation. In the past, I had used yoga essentially as a way to be less stressed and more aware of my daily life. But this stay in Germany offered a striking and stimulating experience, which was particularly inspiring and nurturing.

Every day we woke up at 5.30 a.m. for a first session of yoga meditation, followed by one hour of formal meditation. After that, we would have breakfast together in silence in order to get the day, packed with conference and meditation sessions, off to a good start. As mere amateurs, both Vanessa and I were a bit lost. I was a bit clumsy, and still tend to be, during formal meditation sessions. And yet nothing felt uncomfortable or unpleasant. Just as with the yoga classes, I had the impression that meditation was within my reach; that I could do the exercises in my own way, at my level, without minding the level of those around me. In contrast to many sports or arts, where you need to master certain techniques before you can execute them correctly, for me, meditation is not solely a matter of technique. There is no competitive spirit and there is no need to pitch the level too high. You don't need any equipment or a specific location. And as far as I am concerned, the posture you adopt is not important, nor does it need to conform to the posture of others. What really matters is that you feel well and comfortable. There are no time constraints on carrying out the exercises either. In short, meditation is about a personal journey that each of us can shape to their own liking. What more could one ask for?

Putting words into action, in May 2015 Matthieu Ricard decided to leave his room on the top floor of the Shechen Monastery, near Kathmandu in Nepal, and join my team in Belgium. I welcomed him not only to my lab, but also to my home. He was a real character. Dressed in his Buddhist robe, it was impossible not to notice him – and he certainly caught the attention of my eldest son, Hugo. A year earlier, Hugo had decided to become vegetarian, but I didn't feel ready to prepare special meals, so I had told him that he was too young to do without meat. I confess I also made him believe that not eating meat would seriously jeopardise the growth of his pubic hair. This was all very silly, I admit, but the white lie had worked. When Hugo and Matthieu started to chat over dinner, you could have knocked me down with a feather. Matthieu, a convinced vegetarian, started to encourage my son to become one too, assuring him that what his father had told him made no sense. Moreover, he agreed with Hugo: animals are our friends, so why would we eat them? What's more, Matthieu, as a true scientist, mentioned a good number of epidemiological studies carried out with hundreds if not thousands of subjects, that had established that a vegetarian diet was in fact healthier than a meat-based diet. Ever since, we have all become a bit more flexitarian, which means we try to eat less meat. But Hugo remains our spiritual example as an ethical vegetarian and passionate advocate for animal welfare.

Some people may question whether Matthieu Ricard overdoes it when he's in the limelight. The answer is simple: no, not at all. Matthieu was true to himself each time he came to see us in Liège. He always wore his Buddhist monk's robe, except when he meditated in his pyjamas or bathing suit next to the swimming pool. That is what I admire about him. He travels the world, enjoys a huge following on social media and is adored like a rock star, yet, despite his celebrity, he is very down to earth. He is altruistic to the bone. He is open to discussion on all possible and imaginable topics, even divisive ones, such as karma and reincarnation. He readily questions himself and the Buddhist way of life, and does not hesitate to be subjected to scientific experiments.

The same goes for the Dalai Lama. I know that from experience. Thanks to my collaboration with Matthieu, I was lucky enough to be able to spend a day with him in September 2016. Together with Matthieu and the Dalai Lama, I took part in a conference at the University of Strasbourg on the interactions between science and Buddhism. In between sessions, I had the opportunity to talk with the Dalai Lama, privately and at great length. And he answered many more questions than I had even asked myself. I was surprised at the extent to which he was open-minded and accessible, readily willing to discuss our diverging views about states of consciousness, and the dichotomy between science and religion. Just like Matthieu, the Dalai Lama is anything but egocentric. And when we talked, we addressed each other as 'brother'. Maybe that is why I dared to say to him at the end of the day, 'I don't know if you are a good Buddhist, but I can tell you for sure that you are a good scientist.'

Thanks to the open-mindedness of the Dalai Lama and Matthieu Ricard, I have been able to answer one of my key questions: what effect does

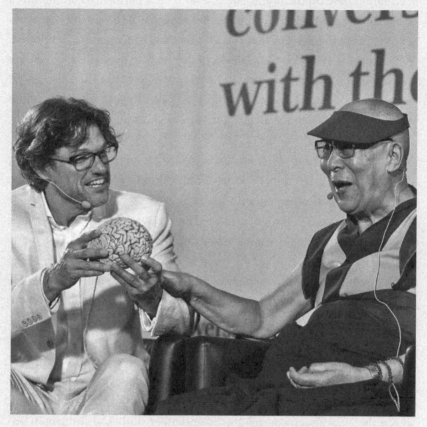

In conversation with the 14th Dalai Lama at a scientific congress
at the University of Strasbourg. © 2016 Olivier Adam.

'My true religion is kindness'

DALAI LAMA

When I asked him what the relation between brain and mind is, the 81-year-old monk replied kindly, 'Our brain is filled with matter that can be measured. That is not the case for our consciousness. There are no material ways that allow us to analyse the mind.' As a neurologist, my aim is to progress our scientific understanding of the mind and the brain, but we can't assume too much. As neuroscientists, it is wiser to say that we can't comprehend how something material like the brain can produce thoughts, perceptions and emotions that are immaterial – in short, our consciousness. It remains one of the greatest mysteries and we are in no position to rule out any hypothesis.

meditation have on the brain? After several tests performed on Matthieu in our lab, we established that his brain is somewhat different to that of his fellow human beings and that certain areas are indeed more developed. When he meditated with over 250 electrodes stuck to his skull, we were able to show that some of his neural networks worked better than the neural networks of others who were, like him, over 70.[1] This is only a fraction of our findings, of which I shall tell you more in this book.

But I can already hear you clamouring! Why is a neuroscientist studying the brain of a master in meditation of interest to us readers? In the same way as studies performed on top athletes help the layman to take up a new running programme, studies performed on meditation experts contribute to our understanding of what meditation can give us all. Like us, many other scientists have studied the brain of meditation experts and, based on their conclusions, others have conducted experiments on lay people and come up with interesting new conclusions that I shall explain in more detail in this book.

Some of these studies are very complex. As scientists, our conclusions very much depend on the equipment we have access to for our studies. What's more, it is impossible to reach conclusions on the basis of just one study, unless there have been control groups and other studies to confirm it. Scientific studies must fulfil a whole series of criteria for the results to be reliable and published in scientific journals. It is a very painstaking process that I shall also clarify in the following pages. Several years of research on meditation have allowed me to accumulate knowledge. I am still a learner in matters of meditation, but as a brain scientist and also a clinical neurologist, I am convinced by the

I hope to convince you that meditation can supplement modern Western medicine.

many published studies that meditation can contribute to better mental health and quality of life. And this is what I would like to share with you. My aim is to encourage you to try meditation and consider it as a preventive lifestyle measure and interesting supplement to modern Western medicine. Hence my rather bold question: why not experience it for yourself? It would seem a shame to refuse to try out new and different avenues, wouldn't it? We live in a world of perpetual mutation. Science doesn't stop, so let's not stop either!

This book aims to demonstrate that there is a supreme path forward, mid-way between the hard sciences, and the more subjective contemplative and spiritual practices. Let's be clear: I don't want you to convert to Buddhism. I did not do so myself. But what I am in a position to do is to give you the tools to better understand why meditation can represent an added value and how you can get started. I hope that in this way you will manage, just as I did myself, to carve your own path in the fabulous world of meditation techniques and brain gym exercises. It is a world without constraints, where nearly everything is allowed as long as you act in full awareness. Take the time to immerse yourself in the knowledge and practice of meditation. Try out the exercises that you find most interesting and discover what meditation means to you.

It is clear that one should always establish clear boundaries between personal opinions, anecdotal situations and scientific studies underpinned by robust data. But I find it a pity that so little attention is paid to the psychosocial and personal aspects of our current medicine. Let's consider the placebo effect. It is an incredible phenomenon that reflects the influence of our mind on our body. The same goes for hypnosis and meditation. And yet these practices are still not always taken seriously. It is clear that we can't cure all illnesses by meditating, but meditation can certainly reduce stress and supplement medication.

This book will not promote a certain form, method or tradition of meditation. On the contrary, what I would like to propose are ways in which you can build your own relationship with meditation. You may spend hours on your mat or simply limit yourself to inhaling and exhaling consciously several times. It doesn't matter. Whatever exercise works for you, it will yield its benefits. Choose whatever suits, according to your needs in the moment. Some Zen traditions, which supposedly recommend that a monk calls you to order with a stick if your posture is not right, would not suit me at all!

I suggest you start with a small experiment. Take a small piece of your favourite (Belgian!) chocolate or make yourself a nice cup of tea. Take the time to look at this treat, to sniff it, to take a deep breath and savour it. Focus entirely on what you're doing and let yourself be carried away by the experience. Now eat the chocolate or drink the tea. What perfumes, what tastes, what thoughts and what feelings do you experience? You'll notice how aware you are of that little piece of chocolate or that cup of tea and how much you like it. I bet that the sensations are much stronger than if you had swallowed the chocolate in one go or gulped down the tea without thinking about it. This is meditation: a simple exercise in awareness. So are you tempted?

~

Chapter 1

Happiness within reach... of your brain!

~

'The secret to happiness is freedom... and the secret to freedom is courage.'
– THUCYDIDES, Athenian statesman, 460–400 BC

Everybody seemingly wants to be happy, to feel cheerful, energetic, in love, relaxed and strong. We all want to enjoy good health, appreciation from our peers and be capable of tranquil wisdom. The question is how to achieve that, given that everything originates in our brilliant brain and mind. My aim is to help you to understand the brain and mind, how they function and how meditation influences them. But let me reassure you, I will not bombard you with either neurological terms or words in Sanskrit – or any foreign language for that matter. I will only share with you some stories, some clinical anecdotes, and some scientific and medical insights, so that you are in a position to understand what happens in the brain, why in all likelihood it functions the way it does and what the consequences of those functions are.

This reminds me of an anecdote. Some years ago, I received an invitation to give a presentation on meditation to a group of teenagers, which I accepted with pleasure. To my great surprise I found myself in front of 130 students who had been waiting impatiently. When I asked them who had experienced stress, worry and insomnia, eight out of 10 raised their arm. Against all expectations, these children were very keen to do meditation exercises with me, whereas I was convinced, probably just as much as you are, that they were leading a peaceful and worry-free existence. Apparently, just like adults, they were in need of a calm and quiet space where they could put their worries aside for a while. I was concerned that, even at their age, these children already had so many worries, and were so much in need of ways to relax and clear their heads.

To think and mull over ideas, is, unfortunately, inherent in our nature! Experiencing an unrelenting flow of thoughts, opinions and analyses is such a ubiquitous phenomenon that we even have a name for it: the 'monkey mind'. The fact that human beings think and are aware that they are thinking is a relic of their evolution from primate to homo sapiens.

Through the centuries, the human brain has been programmed to identify both positive and negative stimuli, both opportunities and threats. This was already the case for the microorganisms that populated the planet. These microbes were equipped with very useful sensors that helped them locate secure places, where they could find food, and thus avoid more dangerous places. This survival mechanism developed according to the evolutionary needs of life on earth. For instance, our prehistoric forebears understood that they could survive by picking wild berries and hunting small animals, and that they should stay clear of larger wild animals. Our brains subsequently developed and became more complex, and fine-tuned this integrated survival mechanism over time.

Our brains learnt to swiftly process all sorts of sensory stimuli, including images, sounds and smells, in order to act rapidly. Let's take a simple example. As you enter the shower, your eyes happen to notice a black spot near the shower drain. In a split second, your brain reviews all the personal experiences it has archived and decides that it may be a spider. As a result, you yell, your pulse accelerates, you start to sweat and you are on the defensive. It took you a split second to step back out of the shower. It's only on closer scrutiny that you come to realise that what you saw were just a few hairs and that there was no reason to panic. Your body relaxes again and you can take your shower peacefully.

This over-developed and fine-tuned survival mechanism is, of course, the reason why we have progressed so far in terms of evolution. But unfortunately, it is also the reason why, in the 21st century, we sometimes over-react and are subject to so many episodes of stress. Our internal survival mechanism has become so complex that our brain is never quiet, even when we are falling asleep at night. How many times have you lain awake because you're struggling with too many thoughts at once? You feel danger lurks round every corner, be it traffic jams or terrorist attacks, not to mention urgent deadlines, the ceaseless fear of the future and of what might happen after the COVID-19 pandemic. Our internal survival mechanism is in overdrive and we can't let go anymore. Literally and figuratively! The area responsible for all this anxiety, which in neurological terms is called 'the internal awareness network', continues to be active even in some comatose patients, a bit like the humming of a fridge that has not yet been disconnected.

In short, our brain is beset by stimuli and we are overwhelmed. This is when feelings of stress, anxiety and depression prevail over pleasant feelings, such as peacefulness and pleasure. Luckily, there is a way out. We are all in the same boat, but we can still cope. The question is how? By reconfiguring our partially pre-programmed brain and, in particular, especially through meditation. I speak from personal experience, but I am also in a position to demonstrate this from a scientific and clincial perspective. Decades of research based on a dialogue between psychology and the neurosciences on the one hand, and the contemplative world on the other, have taught us that meditation is a means to regain control over little voices in our heads that can't stop talking to us. Meditation is a tool that allows us to deliberately choose to stay calm, detached, and to master the constant flow of our thoughts, perceptions and emotions. It can also offer solutions to modern-day problems, such as dealing with stress and stress-related illnesses, anxieties, emotional difficulties,[1] concentration and attention disorders, depression and burn-out,[2] insomnia,[3] chronic pain,[4] immune system disorders, cardiovascular diseases,[5] general lack of wellbeing, and lack of love, understanding and compassion.[6] In other words, by learning to use your brain differently, by rewiring it and by developing certain areas, you will be able to take your happiness into your own hands. The events that make up the stuff of your daily life are of course important, but it is mainly the way you experience them that matters. By just reading this book, you are already taking the first step towards a quieter life that is more serene, more aware and more positive. Your happiness is indeed partially in the hands of your own brain and mind.

By learning to use your brain differently, by rewiring it and by developing certain areas, you will be able to take your happiness into your own hands.

~

Chapter 2

What exactly is meditation?

~

'Meditation aims precisely at softening the mind and
rendering it more manageable, so that you can choose
to concentrate or to relax, and most importantly
to free yourself from the tyranny of torments
and mental confusion.'

— MATTHIEU RICARD

Daisetz Teitaro Suzuki, a great master in Japanese Zen, was invited to an open-air symposium one day. As he sat totally still, his gaze was fixed on a point in front of him. He looked like a statue. The other guests had the impression he was elsewhere, as if he were experiencing a deep trance. But when a gust of wind blew away the whole pile of papers on the table, Daisetz Suzuki was the only one to make a dart to catch them. He was not cut off from the world. He was, in fact, highly concentrated and entirely aware of what was happening around him.

This short anecdote speaks volumes about the enduring misconceptions about meditation. In order to explain what meditation really is and in what ways it can help you, I shall start by clarifying what it is not.

Meditation ≠ origami

The first cliché I would like to dispel concerns the origami postures that should supposedly be adopted during meditation. You have probably heard about the famous lotus position, where you sit crossed-legged like a pretzel, hands on your knees, palms facing upwards, with your thumb and index forming a circle, while you look straight ahead into the infinite horizon. Forget about it! Meditation does not require nor impose an ideal posture. Although the lotus position is a classic position belonging to the Buddhist tradition, it is not compulsory for meditation. You can choose to sit, to lie down, to stand up or to move around. Personally, I prefer to sit crossed-legged on a cushion. I sometimes like to sit on a chair and, occasionally, before an important meeting, I like to sit at my desk and enjoy the wonderful view that I can see from my office on the top floor of the hospital.

Meditation ≠ thinking of nothing

'I can't manage to cut myself off from the world – meditation is not for me.' Nothing is more wrong! The aim of meditation is neither to cut yourself off from the world nor to think of nothing, but, on the contrary, to be extremely focused, even if that lasts for only a few seconds. Meditation teaches you to stay attentive and be more aware of what happens around you by fixing your awareness on an object and opening your mind to all stimuli experienced in the moment. A little further into the book you will learn how.

Meditation ≠ religion

When I met the Dalai Lama, I asked him what in his view was most important: praying or meditating? His answer was clear: 'To meditate, of course,' because otherwise you would not know whom or what to venerate. Buddhism does not have any god to guide you; you need to figure out your own path. The modern forms of meditation that we practise most often today are inspired by Eastern traditions but they have often been adapted to fit Western purposes. Therefore, you don't need to be a Buddhist, Hindu or mystic to reap its rewards.

Meditation can be practised independently of any belief or religious conviction. As far as I am concerned, I consider meditation to be a set of practical tools that help me to lead a better and more aware life. And here is one of my favourite quotes on that matter: 'Meditation is not something you must believe in, it is something you must do.'

Meditation ≠ daydreaming

I am a scientist, so when I hear words or expressions such as chakra, life-energy meridians, astral energy, aura and energetic field, karma, reincarnation or cosmic awareness, I want to know exactly what is meant. In fact, these are not proven concepts that are scientifically defined, but rather metaphors and spiritual or symbolic notions. I believe that the misconceptions and disagreements on meditation stem from the different meanings that we give to these words.

For a scientist, the word energy, for instance, has a very precise meaning, referring to a phenomenon that can take several forms, such as electromagnetic energy, kinetic energy, gravitational or potential energy, nuclear energy and thermal energy. These specific definitions of energy, whether mathematical or physical, differ from energy as it is understood by the biological sciences and psychology, in particular when we speak of mental energy within the mind, or else the cosmic mental energy that allegedly would exist outside the brain. When I discuss these matters with Matthieu Ricard and my Indian or Chinese colleagues, we are always careful to distinguish between those various definitions and meanings. If you are passionate about esotericism, meditation can add an important ritual to your spiritual experience. Because I am attached to scientific common sense, I am the living proof that meditation can also be down to earth and very practical. In short, everyone can determine the degree of spirituality that they want to put into meditation. That is precisely what I like about it. The film director David Lynch formulated it most compellingly when he told me 'The thing about meditation is, you become more and more you.' So you should not have the slightest concern about meditating in ways that suit you and are to your liking.

Meditation ≠ imposed routine

Assuming you're tempted, I personally believe it is best to meditate however and whenever you can, but well-educated professors, like Matthieu, will encourage you to meditate regularly and as often as possible. There is an old Zen proverb that says, 'If you don't have the time to meditate for 20 minutes, then do it for an hour.'

It is best to meditate however and whenever you can.

However, in my view this doesn't mean you need to dedicate that much time to meditation every day or do it in a specific way, space or moment. In that respect, I am certainly not the best example to follow. Indeed, sometimes I meditate every day for ten minutes and at other times I do retreats during which I meditate for hours in a row.

In fact, I may not have the time – or, let's say, I do not take the time – to meditate formally for months. Like many of us, I need to juggle work and family life, and I have a very irregular schedule. At times, I simply don't have the time or the will to do it, but that isn't a disaster. I can't say it enough: meditation is a personal journey that each of us shapes as we see fit. You can practise it where and when you want, in fashions that suit you best. And a few minutes are always better than nothing! Likewise, I am a passionate advocate for 'informal' meditation. At any moment of the day you can inhale and exhale in full awareness several times and thus take a brief break without doing anything special. You may want to reflect on what you are busy doing and enjoy it fully; you may want to observe what you are experiencing without imposing any judgment; or else you may want to take stock of your emotions.

Meditation ≠ set models

The fact that you can meditate as you see fit means, of course, that you need to find out what suits you best. In this book, I shall suggest exercises you can do. Some will suit you, others won't. That's absolutely normal and nothing to worry about. All I would suggest is that you persist until you find the method that you feel totally comfortable with. Be receptive to different

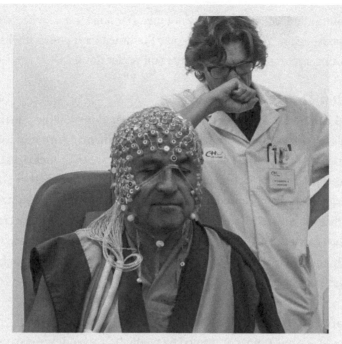

'To consider myself the happiest man in the world makes no sense to me.'

MATTHIEU RICARD

The Buddhist monk Matthieu Ricard is as a guinea pig in our lab. A journalist gave him the title of 'the happiest man in the world'. Here we are trying to measure the activity in his brain in the most accurate fashion, yet, what is he really feeling and what exactly is he thinking?

This is Matthieu engrossed in meditation while we are measuring electrical activity in his brain with an EEG (electroencephalogram) that has more than 250 electrodes. As scientists who are trying to understand human emotions and states of consciousness, we can learn a lot from studying the brains of meditation experts. As he has accumulated more than five years of meditation in solitary retreats up in Himalayan huts, one can safely say that Matthieu is a veritable athlete of the mind. He mainly practises open consciousness, compassion and analytical forms of meditation, as taught by the Tibetan Buddhist tradition. Studying the activity in his brain while he is engaged in different forms of meditation has obliged us to address and overcome many challenges. First, we needed access to state-of-the-art technology in order to measure the activity of billions of brain cells and analyse that activity correctly. (You can discover the detailed results of this study later in the book and in the illustrations on pages 52 and 115.) What's more, I am a scientist and only an amateur meditator. I don't have thousands of hours of meditation under my belt and I am nowhere near being a Buddhist monk, so it isn't easy for for me to understand precisely what Matthieu subjectively experiences during a session of deep meditation. What does he think about? What are his feelings and sensations like? This is a major issue for all studies on matters as personal and individual as meditation, but it is also the case for all studies on the changes in conscious states in general. It goes without saying that we use objective measures, but we need to relate them to what the subject has felt and thought at that moment. This requires intense collaboration and absolute trust between researcher and subject.

possibilities and ask yourself: why not me? The same is true when you take up exercise again. You will need to take the time to ask yourself whether it is running, cycling or swimming that you prefer doing.

Meditation ≠ sects and gurus

What I dislike above all are personality cults that idolise one or several individuals. It is clear that a number of people command admiration, such as Matthieu Ricard and the Dalai Lama. Their lives are their messages, as was the case for Gandhi, Martin Luther King, Mother Teresa or Father Damien. But to let oneself be inspired by them does not mean one follows, trusts or loves them blindly. Meditation also involves knowing how to think critically. Don't get carried away! Trust your instinct and don't follow a guru without questioning what he does. Remain the owner of your own thoughts and the master of your own mind.

Meditation ≠ a practice for specialists

We are all at some point confronted by meditation, even if some of us aren't really aware of it. We tend to forget the capacity to concentrate we developed in childhood, yet to reunite with this form of absorption is a key pillar of mindfulness. One may not always do breathing exercises consciously in the lotus position, but many of us carry out awareness exercises unwittingly on a daily basis. Think of the gourmet who fully enjoys his gastronomic meal, the music lover who is carried away by her favourite piece, or the swimmer who does his laps totally focused. Think of the child you were when you discovered and observed the world with the greatest attention. All are practising mindfulness meditation in some way in that they are extremely aware of what is happening in the moment. Meditation is therefore not only for specialists with mystical rituals and complicated exercises. It is inherent in all aspects of life.

Meditation ≠ reading on topics related to meditation

Books, videos and meditation apps can help you find guidance, information on its benefits, or interesting tips and tricks. So much fascinating stuff has been written on contemplative living that you could spend your whole life reading about it! But it may be wiser to leave all this information aside and focus instead on your breathing. Personally, I have observed that experiencing mindfulness has nothing to do with reading about mindfulness or talking about it with people who do it, just as reading about the last kilometres of a marathon has nothing in common with actually running them. You need to try it out and experience it for your own sake to realise that!

So what is meditation really about?

In order to explain with words what meditation is I shall resort to a comparison. Meditation is like exercise, but a type of exercise meant for the brain. Just like exercise is a common noun for different types of sports, like jogging or bodybuilding, meditation is a common noun that covers different types of mental exercise.

Consequently, just as for exercise, it is possible to choose a certain form of meditation and practise it at different levels. So I consider that the way I do meditation is rather recreational, whereas the meditation practised by Matthieu Ricard places him in a totally different league – that of an Olympic champion. At my level, sometimes a few light physical exercises will do, whereas at other times I may feel the need for an intense two-hour workout at the gym so I can sweat it all out. One day, you may just be happy with a simple informal meditation exercise that lasts no more than a few seconds, but on another day you may feel like doing 20 minutes of thorough exercises of conscious meditation. I find it unfair that those who are sceptical about meditation perceive it to be no more than hype or a marketing trick that allows us to sell books, trendy magazines or overpriced classes. Meditation apps, books and videos are, in fact, rather similar to online jogging and fitness programmes. Of course, it should not be necessary to spend money in order to exercise or meditate, but such tools can come in handy. They are a reminder that training is healthy and they give you a little nudge and feedback to get you going. That is true for both body and mind.

I am not trained as either a sociologist or anthropologist, so it's difficult for me to explain why, in our Western culture, body training became so widespread, whereas there are so many taboos concerning mental training, and psychological or mental disorders for that matter. All too often we consider the mind and body as two separate entities. In reality, they are inherently linked and both deserve our attention.

To meditate is to dedicate attention to the working, the development and the health of one's brain and mind, in order to better understand how it works, and enjoy a feeling of enhanced mental wellbeing and happiness. It is that simple. As a neurologist, my aim in this book is to show how meditation can supplement my medical practice both as a preventative and curative therapy. As a medical practitioner and scientist, I obviously use medication like anti-depressants, tranquillisers and other psychotropic medications when they are necessary, but I have noticed during consultations that my patients tend to ask far too quickly for medication or operations. If they suffer from insomnia, they ask for sleeping pills. If they suffer from stress at work or at home, they request sedatives from their GP. This is a pity, because modern society offers so many other answers or complementary medicine solutions – and I am convinced that meditation and other lifestyle interventions have value.

Understanding that we can gain better awareness of ourselves and those around us, of our emotions, sensations and thoughts, is the first stage of meditation. After that, you will progressively discover the different forms it can take. Indeed, there are an important number of different meditation techniques. In this book I shall give you a thorough introduction to breathing meditation, mindfulness meditation and loving kindness meditation. These forms of meditation stem from Buddhism, but fit in perfectly with our modern Western lifestyles. They don't require you to become a monk or abide by the rules of any philosophical persuasion. And these three meditation techniques are the ones that have been most subjected to scientific scrutiny. That is why we can evidence the benefits they bring and the importance of practising them. And yet, these are only simple methods allowing us to train our brain, to live more mindfully and thus be better equipped to face the stressful situations that life can throw at us.

Mindfulness meditation, for example, is so simple that it can be summed up in just three steps:

1. Find a quiet place and settle in a comfortable position, preferably with your back straight.
2. Focus on a specific object or open your mind to all external stimuli, without letting your thoughts drift. (These two techniques are called, respectively, focused attention meditation and open monitoring meditation, and I explain them in more detail on the following pages).
3. Concentrate as much as possible on the object or the external stimuli.

However, I can tell you now, it is not always that easy! You may lose yourself in your thoughts while you meditate, and that is completely normal. What shall I cook for dinner tonight? Did I change my son's nappy? What time does the meeting start? I am sure you know what I mean. But being aware that you are no longer as focused as you should be doesn't mean that you have failed at meditating. It is even a sign that you have succeeded. As soon as you notice that your thoughts are wandering, you need to refocus your attention on the object in question. It's that simple and that's how easily it is to train your brain.

Apart from mindfulness meditation, there are other kinds of formal meditation. There are several forms of Buddhist meditation, such as Vipassana meditation (insight meditation), Zen meditation (sitting meditation) and, as mentioned above, loving kindness meditation (a form of meditation that encourages positive feelings towards oneself and others). There are also many other forms of meditation stemming from the Hindu tradition, such as mantra and transcendental meditation, in which you focus your attention on the repetition of a word or syllable that doesn't have a meaning, like 'om' or 'rama'. These forms of meditation have enjoyed long-standing popularity with show-biz celebrities – in the 1960s the Beatles became poster boys for the transcendental meditation technique developed by guru Maharishi Mahesh Yogi. Chinese philosophy also offers its own types of meditation, with qigong, a sort of coordinated movement and posture meditation often used for martial arts training, being the most well-known. In our Western Christian tradition contemplative prayer and meditation can also be seen to overlap.

What I am trying to convey is that there is something for everyone. I will take you through the details of three of my favourite forms of meditation: focused attention, when attention can be focused on, for instance, breathing; open monitoring, when you are receptive to all that surrounds you as well as yourself; and, finally, effortless presence.

Focused attention meditation

In this type of meditation, you focus your attention on a single object throughout the session. The object of focus may just be your breathing, a candle you have lit, the sunset, a part of your body, a mantra or a piece of music. As I've mentioned, there is nothing to worry about if you get lost in your own thoughts during this exercise. The fact that you notice it and are able to refocus your attention is part of the exercise. The more you train, the better you will manage to focus your attention, the less absent-minded you will be and the less you will have to fight off the constant flow of thoughts that keeps you from working, disturbs your sleep or drums into your mind. In the long run these exercises can help you to be more focused on a daily basis and have an enhanced capacity of concentration. You will enjoy better control over your state of consciousness, which in turn will allow you to better manage your emotions, your thoughts, your sensations, your stress levels, your pain and your impatience.

Let's do a simple exercise. I am a great fan of meditation focused on breathing and I shall clarify in more detail why a bit later in the book. But here I would suggest that for this first exercise you choose a more concrete and visible object to focus your attention on. This might make it easier for you and will allow for a smoother progress towards the more advanced exercises on offer later in the book.

Seek out a quiet place at home and, as much as you can try, to eliminate any possible source of distraction. Turn off your mobile, the radio and television, shut the windows, dim the lights and turn off all appliances that vibrate, buzz or tumble. Take the time to think of yourself! Place a candle in front of you and light it. Set a timer for two or three minutes. Sit down with your back straight, make yourself at ease and for those few minutes try to focus your thoughts on the flame. If you notice that you get lost in your thoughts, just rid yourself of them and bring your attention back to the little flame. How is it moving? How is the smoke whirling up? What scent are you noticing? How is the candlelight dancing on the table?

Open monitoring meditation

This form is the reverse of focused attention meditation. When you take up this technique, you need to let your mind be receptive to as much as possible in order to register consciously all the stimuli offered by your environment, without judging them or giving them more thought than that. Observation is the operative word. It allows you to intensify your perception of the world around you, as well as your awareness of both internal stimuli, such as your emotions, thoughts and memories, and external stimuli and experiences of the present moment, such as smells and noises. In the long run, it will teach you to live in the present moment and to focus on what happens here and now, to let go of the past and not worry needlessly about the future. As the Vietnamese Buddhist monk Tich Nhat Hanh once said, 'Life is available only in the present moment.'

Let's give it a try together. Sit down in a pleasant place in your garden or next to an open window. Set a timer for two or three minutes and close your eyes. Start listening carefully. What noises are you hearing? Then listen even more carefully. There may be several birds singing or a dog barking as a backdrop to the buzz of the street. Are there children playing or machines humming in the background? Use your sense of smell. Can you identify the scent of damp grass? Or the aroma from the local pizzeria? Or the fragrance of the fresh laundry? Open up to internal stimuli too. What are your feelings? What are you thinking of? What memories and emotions are coming back to you? Let your thoughts roam. Don't try to explain them and don't judge them. Observe them instead and let them float by like clouds in the sky. Are you still getting caught up in thoughts that have nothing to do with the present moment? Divert those thoughts and focus them again on a smell or noise, so that your mind opens up again to the stimuli of the present moment.

Effortless presence meditation

Effortless presence meditation, also called pure being meditation, is less straightforward to explain and is better suited for more advanced practitioners. Often people believe it is about thinking about nothing, but nothing couldn't be further from the truth! When one masters this technique, one becomes fully aware of oneself in the act of meditation. One will have learnt to reach this state of consciousness without needing to focus on a specific object. That may seem a bit vague, but that is the ultimate goal of this type of meditation – transcendence and to reach an enhanced state of 'pure' consciousness, to be aware of one's emotions, sensations, thoughts, the world and those around us, but equally of one's place in the universe and the ways in which it all meshes together and is related.

Now that you understand the distinction between these three meditative techniques, you can try them out for yourself. You will be able to find out what exercises and methods suit you best and experience them through either the exercises on offer in this book, or together with a qualified teacher, a group class, or else with the guidance of the Internet, apps or hightech wearables. If you don't like the first exercise, that's not an issue. Just try the next one. Or, who knows, give it a second chance; the second time round you may reap its rewards. Practice makes perfect, as the saying goes, and perseverance is key to success. Don't set the bar too high, be kind to yourself.

Before I move on to the detailed scientific aspects of meditation and its positive effects on the brain, let me offer a brief recap:

- Meditation is a series of techniques that simply help you train your brain and mind. These techniques can be learnt by all of us, independent of our personality, lifestyle, gender, age, health, our religious orientation or our personal baggage.
- Meditation can help you gain better awareness of your thought processes, emotions, sensations and the world around you. It offers techniques that help you hone your state of consciousness at all levels.
- Meditation is a personal journey that you can shape as you wish.
- Meditation allows you to choose how you want to train your brain to be more aware of what you experience, to become happier and enjoy better health.

~

TESTIMONIAL: SAM HARRIS

'Most of us experience psychological suffering fairly regularly, and meditation is a method of having fundamental insights into that process and finding relief.'

~

Sam Harris is a neuroscientist, philosopher and best-selling author. He also hosts the Making Sense podcast, which discusses the mind, society and current events, and created the Waking Up app which explores the theory and practice of meditation. I had an engrossing and wide-ranging conversation with Sam and here are some of his highly nuanced reflections on mindfulness and meditation.

LANDSCAPE OF THE MIND

How did I get into meditation? In my case, and this is really not unusual, my interest was precipitated by a recreational drug experience. It was MDMA, otherwise known as ecstasy, and I think I was 18. I wasn't at a rave or a party, I took it knowing its potential to reveal something interesting about the nature of my mind. I took it very much in the spirit of investigating my internal universe and seeing what transformative experiences might be on the other side of my ordinary waking consciousness. The experience itself wasn't directly relevant to what I later came to consider the true purpose of meditation, but it revealed for me the fact that it was possible to have a very different experience of myself and the world, my sense of my being in the world, and it was possible to have a much better life than I was going to have by just living out the implications of my own conditioning and tendencies. So it set me on this path of self-enquiry, where I explicitly studied techniques of meditation to try to explore the landscape of my mind further.

I had been given a book by Ram Dass, whose original name was Richard Alpert. Along with Timothy Leary, he had led some of the initial experiments at Harvard in the 1960s, studying LSD. He was also fired from the university, along with Leary, for their misadventures in handing out LSD to all comers. He then went to India, met his teacher, and came back with a very long beard and in a dress, calling himself Ram Dass. He was then a spiritual teacher for many, many years and only died recently. Around 1987 I sat my first meditation retreat with him. He taught an eclectic mix of practices – it was really a kind of buffet of spirituality – including Buddhist meditation, in particular Vipassana meditation. That was the practice I most connected with on that retreat, and then I went on to sit silent Buddhist retreats after that.

I spent a lot of time studying with my friend Joseph Goldstein, who was one of my first Vipassana teachers, and sat with his teacher, Sayadaw U Pandita, a Burmese meditation master. Eventually, I migrated away from strict Vipassana. The logic of the practice, the goal-seeking that was built into it, finally seemed mistaken to me, or at least unnecessary, and was also the source of a fair amount of striving and psychological suffering. Thereafter, I adopted so-called non-dual practices, both within and outside of Buddhism. My approach to meditation shifted significantly, but that took a few years to happen.

So there were several years where I was mostly practising what people in the West know as mindfulness, but very much under a kind of Burmese Buddhist influence, and then I migrated to the Tibetan practice of Dzogchen, but was also influenced by teachers and teachings I encountered outside Buddhism. Meditation practice absorbed a fair amount of time during my twenties. I spent about two years on retreat, having dropped out of Stanford, and I wasn't quite sure how I was going to integrate all these things. Only after that decade, did I return to university to finish my undergraduate degree in philosophy, and then get a PhD in neuroscience at the University of California Los Angeles. It's taken some time, but now I'm in a position to have the kinds of conversations I want to have about the nature of the mind and about what can be understood about it or not, based on first-person methods like meditation.

MEDITATION PRACTICES

I think 'dual' meditation practice is best understood, certainly by anyone who has tried to meditate, by describing the usual starting point for the practice of meditation. So someone decides they want to meditate and they're taught a method. This can be mindfulness or some other technique, perhaps using a mantra or a visualisation. Most of us start that project from a specific point of view. People generally close their eyes, and if it's ordinary mindfulness practice, they might be told to focus on the breath. If you close your eyes and you try to pay attention to your breath, most people will feel that their consciousness is a kind of a locus of attention in the head, which they then must aim at the object of meditation.

Of course, the real obstacle to doing this successfully is distraction, getting lost in thought, and thereby getting pulled away from the object of meditation. You then bring your attention back to the breath, or to a mantra or any other object of attention, and as your concentration builds, this project can become more and more successful. At some point, your attention will actually rest on the object of meditation for longer periods of time. If you're practising mindfulness, you can become good enough to notice thoughts arising as objects, rather than merely being taken away by them in each moment. Many interesting changes in one's mental life can happen here, but if you're practising dualistically, it more or less always feels like there's a meditator on one side — a subject who is paying attention — and the objects of awareness on the other.

As matter of experience, this duality between subject and object is an illusion. And it's the primary illusion that meditation is designed to cut through. If you're practising really well in this dualistic way, the apparent distance between subject and object will occasionally collapse. It may happen a fair amount if you go on retreat and do nothing but meditate for 12 to 18 hours a day, and your mindfulness gets very continuous and effortless. You might find that this subject/object distance collapses again and again and again. You might hear a sound, for instance, and in that brief moment when the sound is impinging on your eardrum, you might notice that there is no sense of one who is hearing the sound. There's just hearing; there's no 'you' in the head listening to a bird out there; there's just this ineffable appearance of hearing that is unified. The subject drops away and the object drops away, and there's just the unity of knowing, but again it's haphazard. You don't have any control over it and when it stops happening you're left thinking, 'Oh, that was interesting. How do I get back to that?' Under that way of practising it seems like the only way back to that is to once again summon an heroic level of concentration and continuity of mindfulness.

ONE UNDIVIDED

What non-dual paths of meditation have understood is that there really is a fundamental illusion to cut through there. It's not the case that you need sustained concentration to get to this experience of unity or non-duality. In fact, consciousness itself doesn't feel like a centre in the head; it doesn't feel like a spotlight of attention being aimed at objects. There is no self in the head, no thinker of thoughts, there's just this open condition in which everything is appearing, and it can be recognised as such directly.

That recognition is the starting point of a non-dual practice like Dzogchen. You can't really begin practising it until you recognise that this is the way consciousness already is, but once you do, then your mindfulness becomes synonymous with that recognition. What you become mindful of is not the breath or sounds or anything else per se, but that there's no subject in the middle of consciousness. The practice itself becomes simply familiarising yourself with this intrinsic property of consciousness that you have basically spent every previous moment of your life overlooking.

So that is the difference. It's somewhat paradoxical to talk about and can be confusing to many people, but I think most people realise that whether they're trying to meditate or not, they do feel like a subject. They don't feel identical to their experience: they feel like they're at the centre of their experience; they're having an experience. They're appropriating it from a place in the head and that's the central illusion that is cut through in non-dual practice.

WHY MEDITATE?

The most common why — the why that is certainly advocated by Eastern traditions generally — isn't really intellectual curiosity. It's much more a matter of overcoming suffering. We all feel unhappy in our lives to some degree or other. That's not to say that happiness doesn't come, but it also goes. You just can't stay joyful all the time, and if you wait long enough, you'll feel frustrated and annoyed and angry and sad and fearful. Most of us experience psychological suffering fairly regularly, and meditation is a method of having fundamental insights into that process and finding relief — so that you don't keep suffering to the same degree and in all the ordinary ways. And it certainly holds out the promise that it might be possible not to suffer at all and to fully escape the logic by which you tend to make yourself miserable. It has a lot to do with having insight into the nature of thought itself and breaking one's identification with thoughts. So much of our psychological discomfort is mediated by our thinking about the past and the future, and failing to connect with the present, because we're thinking so much and not noticing that we're lost in thought.

My motivation for meditating, while it was always somewhat intellectual as well, was primarily about living a better life, in the sense of not suffering unnecessarily and actually being happier, recovering more quickly from the ordinary collisions in life that cause psychological pain. I think that is certainly the most common motivation and for me both of these motivations continue. What's changed for me is that it's not so much a sense of practising deliberately anymore. I do sit and meditate occasionally, but it's much more a sense of always practising. My moment-to-moment experience is always punctuated by what would be meditation if I happened to be in a formal session of practice. This is just a recognition of the way consciousness is, and it happens automatically. It doesn't happen all the time. I spend an impressive amount of time still lost in thought, but when I'm not lost in thought the thing that I am aware of is this non-duality of subject and object in consciousness.

In the beginning, I was trying to achieve this experience, and meditation was a formal attempt to do that. Initially, it was haphazard, and then I could experience it more or less on demand. But now there's much more a sense of 'This is the way consciousness is.' I might inadvertently overlook it, but when I no longer overlook it, it is what I'm restored to in even ordinary moments. So it no longer feels like a practice of any kind. In fact, when one is really meditating, one isn't doing something; one is doing less than one normally does. Meditation is simply the absence of distraction, the absence of being lost in thought for that moment.

THE HUMAN CONDITION
I have had many experiences of intense mental suffering — nothing out of the ordinary, just the usual sorts of suffering that people experience in life. When I was 13 my best friend died. When I was 17 my father died. When I

was 18 my girlfriend broke up with me. These are ordinary experiences. Some people don't have anyone die until they're a little bit older than I was, but if you just wait around, people are going to start dying on you. I was not living in a civil war. There was nothing unusual happening in my life — and all things considered, I had a very lucky life. But those early experiences hit me really hard. For instance, after my girlfriend broke up with me at Stanford, I was probably in some kind of clinical state of depression. For several months after that I was not myself, and it was because I was thinking incessantly about what I had lost — essentially meditating on loss and loneliness and grief. I had absolutely no insight into this process — but, of course, that's nearly everyone's condition.

If you do not see an alternative to being identified with the next emotionally laden thought that arises in your mind — whether it produces anxiety, or anger, or sadness over a loss you've suffered — if there's no space around this automaticity, then there will be no alternative but to live out the emotional implications of whatever this thought happens to be. Most of us, most of the time, have, at best, mediocre thoughts.

UNDERSTANDING THE MECHANICS

We don't tend to tell ourselves a story about how good life is, how grateful we are for all that we have, how beautiful the people in our lives are and how lucky we are to be with them. You can decide to shape your thoughts very deliberately along wholesome lines, and that will improve your mood. This is a very useful practice, and very supportive of mindfulness and these other meditation practices we're talking about, but most of us don't tend to do this automatically. Most of us think about all our disappointments. We notice everything that's wrong in the world. We have a long list of things we want, or wish would happen, and so we tend to be captured by a story of deficiency.

We're telling ourselves a story: if only we could change these things about our lives. If only I could get another girlfriend; or if only I could get back to the girlfriend who broke up with me... It's this idea that if we could only arrange our lives perfectly our attention would rest in the present moment, and we would be satisfied. But unless you have a mind that is capable of real rest, that's not what happens. You get what you want, and you find that you simply want other things.

I'm not saying it's not better to get what you want than to suffer one disappointment after the next. Yes, there are ordinary sources of pleasure and happiness in this life, but none of them are durable sources of happiness. They all tend to degrade. You accomplish one goal, and no matter how wonderful an experience it is, it doesn't take 15 minutes before people start asking what are you going to do next? Nothing gets finally banked as the foundation upon which you can rest and be happy every moment thereafter. Meditation is the practice of understanding something about the mechanics of this cycle of dissatisfaction, and about the search for happiness altogether. If you're running on this hamster wheel, at some level you're not getting anywhere, and the only way to truly come to rest is to deliberately step off it. It may sound trite to say it, but you can't become happy. You can only be happy. Meditation is a method of discovering this truth, again and again.

TEACHING EMOTIONAL WELLBEING

Do we neglect emotional wellbeing in our educational system? Yes, this is something my wife Annaka has focused on a lot. She's taught mindfulness in schools for some years. Initially kids can learn to simply become more aware of what they're feeling. For instance, six-year-olds can recognise specific emotions clearly and see how they motivate them to behave in certain ways.

That's an amazing skill to teach, and it's the first step towards living an examined life – which was so central to Western philosophy for at least a thousand years. And then we lost it, which is why so many people like myself gravitated towards Eastern traditions, because of the value of wisdom – wisdom as opposed to mere knowledge – while never completely disappeared in the West, it got submerged by other priorities.

It has been the case for centuries now that being philosopher in the Western tradition carries absolutely no implication that you're living a better life. There need be no connection between philosophy and wellbeing, or living ethically. Some of the greatest philosophers of the Western canon were just utter neurotics and otherwise toxic human beings. You have someone like Nietzsche, who was profoundly unhappy and seemed personally insufferable. Or Schopenhauer, who threw his housekeeper down a flight of stairs. Or Wittgenstein, who beat pupils and treated his colleagues terribly. These are not people to emulate in terms of how they lived their lives. Obviously, each of them were brilliant and can be profitably read for their thoughts, but there was an important bifurcation between what philosophy became in the West and its original purpose, which was to understand something about the nature of being in the world, such that it transforms your capacities as a person. Philosophy should transform the moment-to-moment quality of your life.

We have largely lost that. It is quite strange that we don't even teach wisdom in our education system and just rely on people to solve the riddle of how to be happy themselves once they become adults. Teaching children to become happier, wiser, more ethical people — I think that's the most important project we have.

~

Chapter 3

A close-up of your brilliant brain

~

'We are all now connected through the Internet,
like neurons in a giant brain'

– STEPHEN HAWKING, British mathematician, physicist and cosmologist

Let me reassure you: there is no need to be a trained neurologist to be able to read this chapter! I just want to share with you some key concepts, since there is a lot of brain activity taking place during meditation. This will allow you to better understand the ways in which neurologists, psychiatrists, psychologists, neuroscientists and myself have come to the conclusion of this book: that the brain probably greatly benefits from meditation.

Everything happens in the mind and hence (probably) the brain

The brain is a jelly-like mass that weighs a bit less than a kilo and half and contains 86 billion neurons or brain cells. These cells transmit and receive all kinds of external and internal information. They are located in the grey matter, i.e. the cerebral cortex, which is the true seat of our cognitive, sensory-motor and emotional faculties. Each neuron involved in brain activity is linked in turn to other neurons through tens of thousands of connections called synapses. Synapses allow neurons to send electrical signals thanks to neurotransmitters. In principle, these chemical molecules can transmit two types of message: 'Hey, do something!' or 'Hey, stop!' Each neuron in the brain sends between one and 20 signals every 10 seconds, so by the time you reach the end of this paragraph, your neurons will have sent trillions of signals. It should come as no surprise, then, that your head is spinning from all these words and figures.

Given its intense activity, the brain uses 20 to 25 per cent of the body's total energy, even though it only represents 2 per cent of its total weight. All these signals are communicated continuously, even during rest or sleep. This phenomenon can be described as 'the mind', 'awareness' or the 'content of consciousness', and it covers not only thoughts, but also sensations, feelings, personality traits, memories, knowledge, desire, dreams, pain and happiness. Everything (or nearly everything) happens in the mind, but in all honesty, no scientist knows how this intense brain activity produces these conscious experiences. We will have to wait for a couple of future Nobel Prize laureates to explain this or perhaps for a fundamental paradigm shift in the key concepts and experimental practices that organise this field of research.

To account for the complexity of our mind and brain and the fact that it never stops emitting signals, several areas and networks have been identified, which, in turn, are associated with very specific characteristics. For instance, when you think intensely before making a decision or when you work on projects, it is the pre-frontal area that is most active. If you are afraid or anxious, then those feelings are associated with a brain network that involves the amygdala, one of two almond-shaped nuclei located at eye level. It thus becomes much easier to describe and understand in what ways mental exercises such as meditation may affect the workings and development of the brain. Contrary to what was thought for a long time, the brain evolves constantly and can be trained, modified and reprogrammed in a manner that is actually quite conscious. In that respect, you are not defined by a cluster of neurons that endows you with a certain predetermined amount of common sense and talent. The way your brain evolves over the years depends on the balance between nature and nurture; that is to say between, on the one hand, your genes, and on the other, your culture, education, training, and the frequency and mode of training of your brain. We now know that nature and nurture are not one: your surroundings and activities can influence and modify the expression of your genes up to a certain point.

The brain is malleable

Let's do a simple experiment. Look straight ahead. Point your finger to the horizon, arm straight and finger in line with your nose. Continue to look straight ahead while moving your finger left or right at more than 60 cm of your nose, i.e. the length of your arm. Your finger then finds itself in the periphery or extremity of your visual field. If you move your finger far enough it will eventually disappear from your visual field and you won't see it any longer. This disappearance is a phenomenon that is less common among a specific group – the hard of hearing. Indeed, because the brain area that normally regulates hearing is not used by those who are deaf, whether since birth or childhood, it has endorsed another function. Their brain thus compensates for the loss of hearing by developing the capacity for sight more prominently than those who hear perfectly well.

This mechanism, by which the brain develops and evolves according to stimuli and influences, is called neuroplasticity – a fancy word for a notion that is not difficult to grasp. The example of the hard of hearing is an extreme one, but it shows that the brain is constantly evolving and mutating. If you break your leg, for instance, and don't use it for a while, the brain area in charge of controlling it will change and get involved in other processes. Neuroplasticity entails not only that certain brain areas

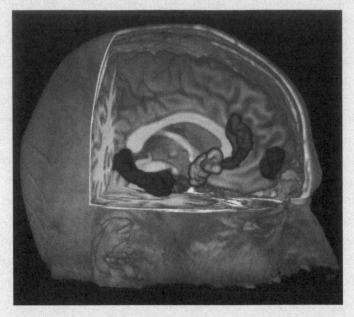

© Steven Laureys

'Happiness is a manner of being and manners can be learnt.'
MATTHIEU RICARD

This is a close-up of the brain of our Buddhist guinea pig, Matthieu Ricard. The brain areas that are most active and developed in experts in meditation such as Matthieu are shown in black in the picture. From left to right: the hippocampus (the darkest black area), the frontal part of the insular cortex (the area in lighter colour), the anterior cingulate cortex (the greyed area) and the prefrontal cortex (located in the front above the eyes).

This picture presents a 3D reconstruction of Matthieu Ricard's head and brain. (Perhaps you will have recognised his face). Let me summarise very briefly the results of dozens of fMRI studies on meditation. The zones that were flagged with extraordinary changes in their functioning and their structure are the following: the hippocampus, key to memory and emotions; the insular cortex, key to the perception and control of internal stimuli, including pain; the anterior cingulate cortex, key to attention and decision-making. More and more studies have shown the effects of lay, i.e. non-religious, meditation on a healthy brain. But there is still a lot that we need to learn about how neurobiological processes underpin meditation and how the therapeutic uses of meditation can help patients suffering from chronic pain, anxiety, depression or other mental conditions, and can supplement traditional medication. Longitudinal studies, i.e. long-term studies, on the brain that monitor a number of patient populations as they learn specific meditation techniques, and compare them with other treatments, will be very valuable in helping us understand the indications, efficiency, contraindication and side-effects of the different therapeutic protocols available, whether in pharmacotherapy, psychotherapy or meditation.[1]

endorse other functions when they are not used, whether temporarily or permanently, but also that certain areas can develop more prominently when stimulated. We have, for instance, observed that with professional pianists the brain areas activated by fine hand-movement are more prominently developed than in the average person. This same phenomenon can be observed in natural-born mathematicians or linguists – polyglots like my daughter Clara, who speaks five languages. When you regularly speak foreign languages or do maths, the brain network in charge of treating the information will indeed be more developed.

Unfortunately, the mechanism cuts both ways and operates negatively too. A person who has suffered several episodes of depression might be more prone to relapse, because the brain network involved has been stimulated more often. In short, neuroplasticity means that the brain is malleable. Reading this book will also change your brain – at least it will if you remember anything of it. Just as it is possible to develop certain muscles by training certain parts of the body, it is possible to develop certain brain networks and connections by practising appropriate mental exercises. This knowledge forms the touchstone of our research on meditation.

Studying the brain and how its working perpetually evolves has been made much easier and more interesting with the emergence, about 20 years ago, of medical imaging equipment, such as fMRIs, PET scans and EEGs:

- fMRI (functional magnetic resonance imaging): this powerful scanner, which takes pictures of the brain, allows us to examine how it is structured and how it functions.
- PET (positron-emission tomography): this imaging technique uses radioactivity to measure the functioning of the brain, for instance when it consumes energy (such as sugar tagged with a radioactive marker) and maps it out.
- EEG (electro-encephalogram): this is a device that serves to measure the electrical activity in the brain with electrodes that are placed on the scalp. It looks like a swimming cap with lots of wires. This equipment allows you to closely monitor to the millisecond the activity in the cerebral cortex. We now have at our disposal equipment that allows us to see directly what is happening in the human brain. We can read on screen the activity and changes that take place in it — after numerous

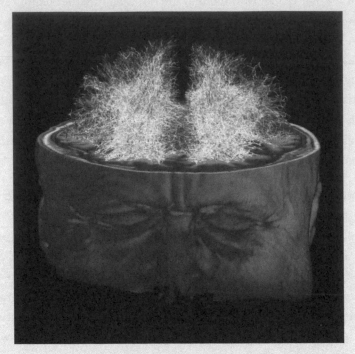

© Steven Laureys, assisted by Sepehr Mortaheb, Engineer
and a PhD student from our team

A better-connected brain is a more efficient brain

White matter — the thousands of billions of brain connections — is also developed to unusually high levels in the brain of our expert in meditation, Matthieu Ricard, compared with other 70-year-olds who enjoy good health, but do not meditate.

One can see in Matthieu's brain an increased level of connections between the two hemispheres, in particular in the bridge located in the middle of the brain behind the nose. Studies would seem to show that the efficiency of this connection between the two hemispheres becomes more salient as the meditation experience intensifies.[2]

and complex calculations and statistical analysis, I grant you that. It's a bit like Disneyland for neuroscientists. All the more so, when we had the opportunity to observe the brain activity of Matthieu Ricard. So why is it so interesting? In order to improve, one must seek out the best of the best. In order to cook well, you may pick up good ideas by watching a cookery programme on TV. To learn to play chess, it can't harm to study a Garry Kasparov video. To know how meditation improves the brain, it may help to observe the brain of a monk such as Matthieu. It is that simple!

Obviously, it wasn't always a picnic in the park for Matthieu. Imagine having to lie still for hours on end in a scanner while scientists who are curious about your brain give you all sorts of absurd instructions. 'Please blink less because it can distort the results' or 'Go into deep meditation. We will at some point make a loud bang to examine your startle reflex.'[3] Matthieu had a couple of dozen electrodes and a big magnet attached to his scalp. The latter pounded continuously against his skull while he was meditating on demand. Hats off to the man, who bore this hammering without ever complaining. However, the eventual results were significant and when supplemented by, and analysed with, other similar studies, we were able to expand the boundaries of our knowledge of the power of the mind and meditation.

Close-up of Matthieu Ricard's brain

What can be observed in the brain of a seasoned expert in meditation who has thousands of hours of mental training under his belt? We can say without doubt that intensive training in contemplative practices does affect the brain. If you believe that meditation is just a waste of time, I would invite you to reconsider your view and delve into Matthieu's cranium. You will be able to see the significant influence not only on the structure of his brain – more grey matter – and on its connectivity – more white matter – but also on the brain activity itself. We now know that mind training and muscular training have something in common. Muscles can be enhanced and developed thanks to targeted exercises. Likewise it can be seen that Matthieu's brain has developed thanks to targeted mental exercises.[4] Practically speaking, we have observed the thickening of his grey matter in the brain areas involved in concentration (the prefrontal cingulate cortex), in internal regulation (the insular cortex and amygdala) and in memory (the hippocampus).[5] Matthieu has produced these changes by doing numerous meditation exercises.

Neurons, which constitute the grey matter, differ from other types of cells as they are characterised by their interconnections. The brain consists of billions of neurons and the number of interconnections between those neurons can reach 100 trillion – at least 10,000 times the number of stars in our galaxy. A healthy brain is a well-connected brain in which all areas can exchange information swiftly. The speed of information transmission depends on the white matter. With people like Matthieu we find higher levels of connectivity, thanks to more bands of myelin, a fatty white substance that sheathes and isolates neurones, and allows them to send information more efficiently and quickly in the form of electrical signals.

To conclude, one can say that Matthieu has a particularly well-preserved and well-connected brain for a man over 70. If we compare brain connections to a motorway network, Matthieu has several additional lanes and better control of traffic density. But let's not linger on the feats of a single meditator, especially since studies carried out on dozens of experts have all shown similar results with little variations between individuals. The important point here is that differences are mainly due to the training itself, rather than the extraordinary qualities of one Olympic champion-like[6] individual.

As well as the structural changes in Matthieu's brain, thanks to the fMRI tests and EEGs we also identified intensified levels of activity. We also noted a certain a stability, which means less uncontrolled mind-wandering in comparison with the layman. Such a degree of thought mastery is not unique to Matthieu. It can also be observed in Lama Zeupa, with whom I did a four-day retreat. A previous study, led by Antoine Lutz and Richard Davidson[7] at the University of Madison, looked at how compassion meditation affected the brain during one meditation session with Matthieu and about 15 other experienced meditators. It found an unprecedented high frequency of gamma waves in his brain and also identified stronger activity in the left area of the prefrontal cortex compared to the right one. This has been interpreted as a very developed capacity to experience positive feelings (when people are depressed it is often the contrary that happens) and a reduced tendency to negative thoughts.

If we compare brain connections to a motorway network, Matthieu has several additional lanes and better control of traffic density.

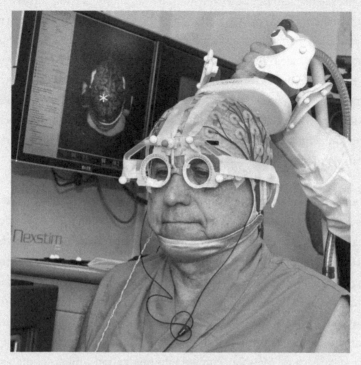

Matthieu Ricard and our team of collaborators contributed
to a world premiere at our GIGA Consciousness Research Unit © 2015 University Hospital Liège

'Meditation consists in freeing the mind'

JIDDU KRISHNAMURTI, INDIAN PROPHET, 1895–1986

We asked Matthieu to enter into deep meditation while we actively stimulated certain areas of his cerebral cortex using powerful magnetic waves, emitted by the white mallet-shaped device placed on his head. He was wearing a cap equipped with sensors that measured his electrical brain activity on a constant basis. The strange glasses, the sensors on his cap and the magnet allowed us to know precisely which part of the brain we were stimulating. You can actually see it on the screen behind his head, where it is shown with a star. It was not very pleasant for our guinea pig and that shows in his facial expression, but it allowed us to objectively evidence the impressive power of meditation over the ability to control the mind as well as the working of the brain. This had never been done before. After the first measurements taken with Matthieu, we decided to do further tests with other subjects. But given the exceptional and unexpected nature of our observations, the results we obtained with Matthieu were published as a case study in a scientific journal. Dr Ricard, of course, appeared as co-author.[8]

To date, science had not been able to make such observations. This earned Matthieu the accolade of 'happiest man in the world', although the journalist was sensationalising the study and it was about compassion not happiness. In fact, as Matthieu himself pointed out, it is impossible to reduce happiness to a brain measure since it is a mode of being that results from various human qualities, compassion and kindness among them. 'How could one possibly know the state of mind of more than seven billion human beings? These kinds of statements are nice and well-intended, but slightly naïve,' he commented.

But what is a gamma wave exactly? It is a very high frequency wave produced in the brain when, for instance, you bite into an apple consciously and all senses, including taste, hearing, smell and sight, are activated. The electric activity in the brains of Matthieu and his colleagues reveal a greater presence of gamma waves, whatever task they perform. The increase in gamma waves in those who practise meditation seems to be proportionally higher according to the length of meditation practised and the estimated number of hours. This made it difficult for us as scientists to define a reference state, because Matthieu entered into meditation almost spontaneously and we needed to encourage him actively not to be mindful or to meditate.

Our research team made some amazing discoveries by studying Matthieu Ricard's brain close up.[9] We examined how, by using a magnet to disturb his brain activity, we could modify and measure its electrical activity at the same time. This test is normally used to evaluate the brain's level of consciousness in a clinical setting. This is particularly useful when one seeks to measure the mind of a comatose or anaesthetised patient, for instance. Thanks to the power of meditation, Matthieu was the first person to be able to influence this test, voluntarily increasing and decreasing his functional brian connectivity and consciously controlling his content of consciousness and measured functional brain connectivity. Not everyone can do this, only meditation champions can. This capacity needs to be explored further with a larger group of experienced meditators.

Understandably, these tests were not always pleasant for Matthieu. He had to remain sitting still without moving, with strict instructions to go into deep meditation while his brain was being mechanically pounded. Yet he always remained friendly and obliging, as only the happiest man in the world could be. When we asked him to go for different states of meditation, he chose loving kindness meditation, compassion, focused attention and mindfulness or 'open presence', to use his own term. I also asked him at some point to reduce his conscious awareness and go into a sort of 'zombie state'. Even though that is not the aim of Buddhist meditation, which seeks to cultivate a calm but clear mind, Matthieu tried to enter the most reduced cognitive state. He took up the gauntlet with good humour, calling this type of meditation 'self-induced cognitive opacity'. He told us that he imagined himself being totally immersed in a mud bath, with thoughts emerging from time to time, like little bubbles that dissolve right away. It is true that it is impossible 'to think of nothing', even for Matthieu Ricard. There will always be minimal brain activity. However, and this is rather extraordinary, he managed to enter a pseudo-comatose state very quickly. Apparently, Matthieu is not only able to control his thoughts and emotions, but he is also capable of influencing the level of clarity of his consciousness and the complexity of his brain activity, as our equipment evidenced.

The brain in full meditation mode

It goes without saying that we don't all have it in us to meditate for more than 60,000 hours, as Matthieu has, yet it isn't necessary either. Neuroscience has explained how our experiences determine, to a certain degree, what our brain physically looks like, and this is the neuroplasticity, which I referred to earlier.[10] In cases of chronic stress, for example, we see changes in how the amygdala functions. Certain events that occur during the first years of life have a particularly strong influence on the structure of the brain. Newborn babies and toddlers who grow up in a stressful environment may see their brain develop less. Luckily, positive structural and functional modifications can be brought about in the brain as well, thanks to training, cognitive behaviour therapy and certain forms of meditation. As part of a longitudinal study carried out with meditation beginners who had all followed an eight-week course in mindfulness meditation, fMRIs revealed that the participants had less

It is possible to control your own psychological wellbeing through mental training.

grey matter in their right amygdala, which could be interpreted as being due to less exposure to stressful experiences or a heightened capacity to handle them.[11] The results of the ReSource Project led by Tania Singer at the University of Berlin are even more convincing. They evidence changes in neural networks according to the type of meditation, whether mindfulness, perspective-taking or altruistic love.[12] This means that it is possible to control your own psychological wellbeing through mental training. If you decide to take charge of your health by taking more exercise, why not take charge of your mental wellbeing by training your brain? Meditation is no magic wand, but certain types of exercise can modify the structure of your grey matter and their connections, and therefore benefit your social, emotional and psychic life.

The brain during focused attention meditation

We already know a bit more about the effects of meditation on the brain, but what really happens during mindfulness meditation? Scientists at Emory University in Atlanta have carried out fMRI[13] tests on a group of experienced practitioners of meditation in order to observe the mind while it is devoted to focused attention, a meditation exercise during which the mind focuses on, for instance, one's breathing rhythm. The participants were instructed to press a button each time their thoughts wandered. In this way, the team could detect the brain areas that were active before, during and after mind-wandering. They discovered that different neural networks were activated during meditation. In fact, what can be observed is the existence of a cognitive cycle that comprises four phases, which each activate a different network:

1. Mind-wandering

Even Matthieu and the most trained Buddhist lamas have thoughts that wander at some point or another. The famous 'default mode' network then springs into action. This is the fallback network, which comprises the zones that are active 'at rest' – a state during which the brain is not focused on external sensory events – in particular, the median prefrontal cortex, cingulate cortex and the precuneus.

2. The person realises their mind has wandered

When this happens, it is the 'salience' network that comes into play. This involves the brain areas that are always activated when a new event or an event that merits our attention occurs. It comprises areas such as the insular cortex and the prefrontal cingulate cortex.

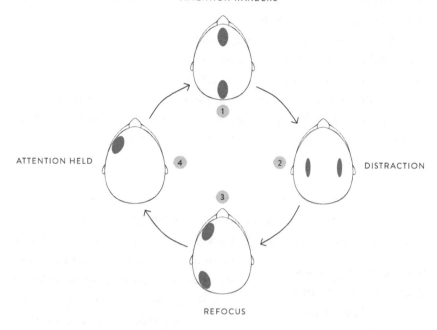

ATTENTION WANDERS

ATTENTION HELD

DISTRACTION

REFOCUS

Meditation is not about thinking of nothing. When you do focused attention exercises, you will learn to observe your thoughts, let them wander and then refocus on your breathing or another object. These exercises activate different areas of the brain and allow you, once you've done them several times, to maintain a higher and more stable level of attention and concentration.[14]

3. The person refocuses their thoughts

Two zones are activated when you refocus your attention on your breathing rhythm or any other object you are concentrating on: the dorsolateral prefrontal cortex and the inferior parietal lobe.

4. The person maintains their attention

When you manage to concentrate all your attention on your breathing or on any other object you are concentrating on, it is the dorsolateral prefrontal cortex that remains active.

This cycle may only take a few seconds. The more experienced a meditator you become, the less this cycle will occur during your sessions. Meditation sessions require less effort on the part of experts in order for them to stay focused. This study, however, has brought up key evidence that mind-wandering is not a bad thing per se, but rather an essential step in the meditation process. It's a bit like the weights you add to your body-building bar: you need a certain 'resistance' in order to ramp it up. Consequently, without mind-wandering, without any distraction and without a mind that at times thinks of something other than, say, breathing, if that is what you are focused on, it is impossible to train your focusing skills and to meditate 'well'. If, when meditating, you suddenly find yourself thinking of your work, your children, your pets or an errand you have to run, don't be disappointed. Stay positive and be happy about it: it is the occasion to train and develop better concentration.

Whether you meditate or not, when your thoughts are not focused on the present moment because you are daydreaming, thinking of something else, worrying or simply letting your thoughts wander, the default mode or fallback network is activated. Expert practitioners in meditation seem to have reduced and different activity in this network.[15] Their minds wander less during their daily activities. Do they benefit from that? The answer would be yes if you read the revolutionary study carried out at Harvard University and unambiguously titled 'A Wandering Mind is an Unhappy Mind'.[16]

Mind-wandering is not a bad thing per se, but rather an essential step in the meditation process.

The research team contacted over 2000 volunteers via a smartphone app either at chosen or random moments to ask them how they felt, whether they were happy, what they were doing and whether they were thinking about the activity they were engaged in – i.e. the present moment that matters so much in mindfulness – or about something else – i.e. past worries or anticipating future imagined events.

The results were really enlightening. Half of the time, we seemingly don't think about what we are doing. Apparently 47 per cent of the participants were spending their time daydreaming. They seemed happier when they were having sex, exercising or were talking to someone else. They were far less so when they were resting or working on the computer. Yet what this study surprisingly concluded was that it was not so much the activity they were carrying out, but rather their state of mind that determined the levels of happiness participants experienced. Only very little of their sense of wellbeing could be attributed to a specific activity, whereas their mind-wandering and ruminations would seem to make them more unhappy. Next time when your thoughts go astray during a conversation with your partner or while you are working on a project with a colleague, remember that another brain network will be called into action and that consequently this mind-wandering, or worse, these ruminations, might seriously jeopardise your sense of enjoyment.

Far too often we tend to differentiate between what we want to do and what we actually do. Yet, when we get rid of the gap between our expectations and actions, our energy focuses on what we are doing in the present moment. Let's not waste our energy on what we think we should have done or what might possibly happen in the future. The secret is to do one thing at a time. Let's do what we do when we do it. 'When you are walking, you are walking.' It is that simple and powerful.[17] Enjoy the pleasures of mono-tasking...

~

Chapter 4

To all those who are impatient and highly sceptical

~

'You will never become brave if you have never been hurt. You will never learn if you have not made any mistakes. You will never succeed if you have never failed.'

AUTHOR UNKNOWN

Before delving into your own mind and getting started with meditation, I would like to address the critical judgement that you all might have. You won't be the first person to question whether scientific research on meditation is reliable. I would therefore like to clarify how we study meditation, the scientific problems we may run into and the ways we try to tackle them.

The British journalist and writer Malcolm Muggeridge once said, 'Never forget that only dead fish swim with the stream.' I don't consider myself a dead fish. As a scientist, if you want to acquire new knowledge, you need to dare by swimming against the stream. This means that sooner or later you will need to face headwinds and the possibility that your work may be classified as a 'soft science' by some colleagues. The expression 'soft sciences' is used to describe scientific studies of which the precision, methodology or purpose is difficult to verify. The cognitive sciences, psychology and sociology, are often considered to be soft sciences. Many scientists who are sceptical, or just cautious, and typically do pure research in animal cellular biology, for instance, will often ask me why I put my reputation on the line as a coma specialist in order to study a topic as 'soft' as meditation or hypnosis. The answer is simple. I am convinced that it is possible to provide scientific evidence for the benefits of the psychological modifications and changes in states of consciousness that meditation and hypnosis produce.

The fact that scientists cannot produce studies underpinned by substantial objective data overnight is no good reason to despise or disparage meditation. History – as does my own scientific journey, by the way – tells us that considerable effort and strategy are required in order to expose, check, double-check and disseminate new knowledge and insights across the scientific world.

In this respect, there is no more striking and extreme example than the discovery of the relation between the Sun and the Earth. In 260 BC Aristarchus of Samos, a Greek astronomer and mathematician, maintained that the Earth revolved around the Sun. Most of his contemporaries thought he was mad. They would not believe that the Earth was moving. It was only in 1728, that is to say 20 centuries later, that it was possible to prove that the Greek astronomer had been right all along. Thanks to the use of a telescope,

James Bradley, an English astronomer, was the first to provide evidence that stars travelled and the Earth rotated around the Sun.

This story is a stark reminder that as a scientist you are only the child of your own times. Your work is limited by the measuring instruments of your era. Step by step, or rather study after study, you nevertheless lay down the foundations of what may one day become a revolutionary insight. And, of course, being able to swim against the stream and face criticism is just part of the game, which, incidentally, has not put off my research teams. We also had to face headwinds when we carried out our research on the states of consciousness of comatose patients, on near-death experiences and the changes in perception under hypnosis, all of which we have been working on for many years. But our teams never stopped fighting – and rightly so! The scientific evidence brought to the fore by these three studies has now proven to be irrefutable.

As far as meditation goes, I believe we are on a similar track. Although we still have a lot of work ahead of us, and our studies need to be developed further, we are gaining in assurance and confidence. But don't get me wrong. As a scientist I remain realistic and cautious. I question all I read and hear about, and am critical of my own work. I won't deny, either, that a substantial number of studies on meditation, as is the case in other scientific areas, by the way, are not sufficiently underpinned by evidence, are published without having been adequately peer-reviewed, and still present many questions. All the more reason to separate the wheat from the chaff! Criticism doesn't only come from the scientific community, but also from Buddhist and religious groups, who aren't always keen to take part in this type of research. That is a pity because the collaboration between the sciences and contemplative traditions has already yielded fascinating results for both camps, and our teams have gladly contributed to these results, regardless of whatever challenges or obstacles they encounter.

As a neurologist, when I look at pictures of brain haemorrhages, I can clearly identify where the problem is located and what repercussions it will have for the patient. To understand this, I don't need to have had a brain haemorrhage myself. It is an objective piece of data that I can read on screen. But when I am with a patient who suffers from headaches or stress, it is not that obvious. Only the patient knows the pain and emotions he is feeling. As a doctor, I can only listen to him carefully and ask him targeted questions in order to establish an appropriate diagnosis on the basis of his explanations and supplementary clinical examinations, in order to exclude certain pathologies. But I won't see the pain and stress represented on an image. Therefore, this data is less objective.

Obviously, one can argue that I have also suffered headaches, but the fact remains that the way my patient describes his pain is more subjective than the scan of my patient who suffered a brain haemorrhage. And so it goes for research on meditation too. Our team was lucky enough to study an experienced master in meditation such as Matthieu Ricard with the benefit of high-tech equipment. We have thus been able to take pictures of the structure and workings of his brain, which has allowed us to visualise in black and white what the brain of an expert in meditation looks like and how it functions.

However, when I asked Matthieu what he was feeling when he meditated and what changes he observed in his own life, his answers were much more personal and subjective, and therefore harder to grasp. As a Buddhist monk, he would at times use terms which were beyond me. When Matthieu talks about 'letting go entirely of his own ego' or about 'reaching a state of pure consciousness,' I admit that I find it hard to see exactly what he means. Matthieu, therefore, is a bit like the patient suffering from headaches who can only express himself within the boundaries of his vocabulary and mine, his experience and mine. This is the second challenge that we face in our research on meditation, and this challenge is all the more substantial, since we want to broaden the scope of our research and progress from studies focusing on masters in meditation such as monks to studies involving larger populations of meditators and non-meditators.

Finally, as part of our research we want to show how meditation and mindfulness can be useful for the layman like you and me, but also for young children, in our educational system; in professional settings; and in the elderly. At present, the challenge is to collect data concerning the subjective experience of a large number of guinea pigs in the most objective way possible. That requires a lot of work and coordination, yet, again, our research team has been up to the task and has succeeded in navigating their way through different pitfalls. To show you that the currently published studies I am using to underpin this book are reliable, I shall start by giving you an example of the difficulties met by those who pioneered the scientific study of meditation.

Back in the 1970s, Dr Daniel Goleman, an American psychologist and member of the steering committee of the Mind & Life Institute, studied the different reactions to stress in a group of 30 amateur meditators and a group of 30 expert meditators while they were watching a violent horror movie. The heart rate and perspiration of the participants were measured from the start of the movie. At first sight, the results obtained by Dr Goleman seemed reliable. It would appear that the stress level of the expert meditators returned to normal much more quickly than those of the group of amateurs. Thanks to these results, Dr Goleman gained his doctorate at Harvard University and these findings were indeed very interesting. However, his results did not necessarily prove that the effects observed could be attributed only, and first and foremost, to meditation. Expert meditators usually have a very different lifestyle to amateur meditators; they have different eating habits and resting routines. Dr Goleman was probably also unwittingly influenced by the participants and it may have been that he was not impartial when analysing his measurements. Nearly 50 years later, our take on this study has changed, as the results of a single study can't provide absolute certainty. Nor can these results be considered to be reliable unless several independent research teams have carried out controlled randomised double-blind studies yielding similar results that prove identical after careful overall analysis.[1]

The process, therefore, demands multiple verifications and considerable work, but respecting this strict research protocol allows us to reach much more convincing results. I'm not the first scientist to meticulously scrutinise a Buddhist monk as experienced as Matthieu Ricard. Our research represents only a very small piece of a much larger puzzle consisting of many years of research. This is why we are now in a position to conclude with much greater certainty that meditation can be beneficial for the brain, for our capacity to focus, for our emotional wellbeing and mental health. There is still further research that needs to be carried out, but the hypothesis that meditation is positive for the majority of us is now solidly corroborated. It should be noted, though, that meditation can be used in less benevolent contexts, as is the case in the American Army for instance, where it is

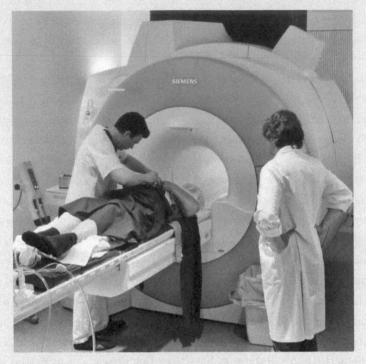

Matthieu Ricard disappears into our MRI scanner so that his brain can be analysed objectively by our team of neuroscientists © 2015 CHU Liège, Brain Centre

'To measure is to know and to guess is to err'
PROVERB

Here we are evaluating to what degree Matthieu, a Buddhist monk who is highly trained and has meditated for more than 60,000 hours, displays signs of changes in his cerebral cortex, i.e. the billions of brain cells or neurons that compose our grey matter. Over the last 20 years, hundreds of MRI studies on meditation, mindfulness, yoga and other mind-body exercises have been carried out. In this book, we are using the results of the measurements taken with Matthieu to illustrate current knowledge about the effects of meditation that has been published in the scientific literature and what stills need to be evidenced. Experts in meditation have a cerebral cortex and brain connections that are highly developed, yet this does not mean you need to become a Buddhist in order to benefit from the positive effects of meditation on the brain and on health in general. Studies have shown that meditating for 20 minutes a day over a course of eight weeks allows you to feel the positive effects on your emotions and behaviour, and that these will already be reflected in apparent changes in the structure and functioning of the brain, in particular in the prefrontal cortex, cingulate cortex, insular cortex and hippocampus. The brain is malleable and evolves constantly.[2]

used as a 'tool to develop soldiers' resilience'[3], in schools to breed students who are 'calm and docile', or in businesses to improve productivity without taking into account employees' wellbeing.

To Dr Goleman's credit, the measuring instruments he had access to as a researcher in the 1970s, particularly for his study, were far less refined than the equipment we use today in our labs. For the first time in history, we can observe the brains of experts and newcomers to meditation thanks to sophisticated pieces of equipment such as fMRIs, metabolic PET scans and high resolution EEGs.

These devices allow us to monitor live what happens inside the cranial cavity when subjects practise different forms of meditation and to compare them with an active control state. Thanks to brain scanners we are now in a position to study how the brain, observed in groups of amateur meditators, changes throughout a standardised and repeatable meditation protocol. We have thus laid the foundations for carrying out a larger-scale study with larger pools of subjects, a study that will in turn show the benefits of meditation for people like me and you. It is therefore necessary to continue developing our knowledge and insights into meditation in order to better understand how it functions, what its benefits or associated risks are, and to gain a critical view on the matter.

It is important at this stage to pay tribute to those who courageously pioneered this research on meditation: the French neurobiologist of Chilean origin, Francisco Varela,[4] the psychologist Richard Davidson at the University of Wisconsin, Madison,[5] and the neuroscientist Clifford Saron at the University of California,[6] as well as the American molecular biologist Jon Kabat–Zinn, who created the Mindfulness–based Stress Reduction (MBSR) programme.[7] Although they were first active 30 years ago, they continue to inspire the community of researchers who work in what is now termed the 'contemplative neurosciences'.[8] To mention just a few, this community includes people such as the American psychologist Paul Ekman,[9] the neuroscientist Amishi Jha,[10] and my neuroscientist friends Antoine Lutz in Lyon, and Tania Singer in Berlin, who have conducted the largest longitudinal study on the topic.[11] As for our own research, we started it with Buddhist monks in 2015 and it continues today thanks to collaborations with other experts, but also with newcomers, and focuses on meditation, hypnosis, trance and other states of modified consciousness.[12]

But let's come back to our first experiment with Matthieu Ricard. Back then, we tried to answer two main questions: 1. What is the effect of the longstanding practice of meditation on the brain? 2. How does the functioning of the brain change during different types of meditation? For this book I again used my favourite guinea pig, Matthieu, to showcase what we think we understand about the effect of meditation on the mind and the brain[13] (see page 55). When he came to my lab at GIGA-Consciousness and the Centre du Cerveau (Brain Centre) at the University of Liège for this new adventure, we used all the equipment at our disposal to study the functioning and structure of his brain, and compare them with other individuals of his age group. The MRI allowed us to measure the volume of both his grey matter, i.e. the billions of nerve cells or neurons, and of his white matter, i.e. the nerve connections or axons (see the illustrations on pages 50 and 52), whereas the fMRI, the PET scan and the EEG allowed us to evaluate functional changes, his oxygenation levels, his consumption of sugar and electric activity. But it is thanks to a cerebral connectivity measurement tool called TMS-EEG (a combination of transcranial magnetic stimulation and an electro-encephalogram) that our team veritably broke new ground.[14] This test consists of stimulating a specific part of the grey matter with a powerful magnet and simultaneously measuring the complexity of the electrical reaction in the rest of the brain. I should add that our team uses this technique at the hospital, in particular in intensive care and neuro-rehabilitation, in order to better measure the levels of consciousness in people who fall into a coma after serious brain injury.[15] This test rests on a theory of consciousness developed by Italian psychiatrist Giulio Tononi at the University of Madison, according to which cerebral information needs to be integrated in order for there to be a conscious thought or sensation.

Without going into too much complex technical or mathematical detail, we can safely say that Tononi's team (Wisconsin), Massimini's (Milan) and our own at Liège (led by Olivia Gosseries) have all demonstrated that this consciousness level test is very robust. It has reliably established that the complexity of the responses we obtain only changes with subjects who are in a coma, under general anaesthesia or in deep sleep. In the other cases, the responses we measure could never have been influenced by the mere will of the hundreds of volunteer participants we have studied.[16]

And then Matthieu came to the lab and revealed how potent the mind of a very well-trained Buddhist monk can be. He revealed for the first time how it is possible to influence these measures consciously and by the power of will only. We studied this phenomenon over several sessions: the baseline condition, i.e. simple rest, during sleep, during open monitoring meditation and finally self-induced opacity meditation, i.e. a state of almost no thought that experts are exclusively able to reach. Such results had never been obtained before in any lab in the world. They were so impressive that the scientific article we then published was limited to reporting, after multiple verifications, the unique case of monk Ricard.

Like other experts in meditation, Matthieu has developed an exceptional level of mental control, but it remains important to understand that, even if studies such as ours have made it possible to establish and test new hypotheses in the field of meditation, everyone can, if they wish, discover for themselves the benefits of meditation and mindfulness on their brain and health. As I've said, there is no need whatsoever to become a Buddhist monk to benefit from the exercises and mental training provided by meditation!

~

TESTIMONIAL: DAVID LYNCH

'If you're a human being you've been gifted with a nervous system that's built for this and it will work.'

~

David Lynch is a filmmaker, actor, artist and musician, perhaps best-known for directing the movies Eraserhead, The Elephant Man *and* Blue Velvet, *and the TV series* Twin Peaks. *He is also a long-term Transcendental Meditation practitioner and in 2005 he founded the David Lynch Foundation for Consciousness-Based Education and World Peace. Since then, the foundation has brought the Transcendental Meditation technique to more than 500,000 children and adults around the world, including disadvantaged young people in inner cities, veterans with post-traumatic stress disorder, and women and children who have survived violence and abuse. I was honoured that he found time to talk to me about Transcendental Meditation and to convince me of its benefits.*

TRUE HAPPINESS LIES WITHIN

I've been doing Transcendental Meditation for 46 years. I had heard a phrase — 'True happiness is not out there, true happiness lies within' — and this phrase had a ring of truth to it for me. I started thinking about the phrase, but it upset me, because they don't tell you where the within is, nor do they tell you how to get there. I believe there's happiness inside somewhere, but how do you get it? So I started becoming a seeker. I started looking into all different kinds of meditation, and I would listen and I would read, and I would say, no that doesn't sound right.

Then my sister, who happened to call me one day, had started Transcendental Meditation. I listened to what she said about it and I liked it, but also I heard a change in my sister's voice. I heard more self-assuredness and happiness in her voice. I put that together with what she told me about it and I said I want that. I went and got it, and I've never looked back. When you're taught you're given the mantra and you're taught how to use it. My teacher took me into a little room. She said sit comfortably in the chair, close your eyes and start the mantra, just as I told you, and I had my first meditation.

I had a great experience with my first meditation. Others, my friend Mario, for instance, he went months without that experience, but then it happened. So the human being has the most incredible nervous system, built for transcending. We've just lost contact with that deepest level. If you picture Transcendental Meditation as gold coming in, garbage going out, and the gold that comes in, you keep it. It doesn't dissipate. In the real world we get happy about something new, something we desire, but a year later we've forgotten about that happiness, we're on to something else. The happiness that comes inside with transcending every day you keep, and it grows, and life becomes better and better each day that we transcend.

FIND A TEACHER
You can still do mindfulness or Buddhism, whatever you want. Just add this technique to your life and you'll zoom forward. You do whatever kind of meditation you want. I'm not here to tell you anything about what you should do, but it's a real change that happens because of transcending every day. My advice to you is to get a legitimate teacher of transcendental meditation as taught by Maharishi Mahesh Yogi. You will get this technique, and you will sit down and have a meditation. If you are a human being, it will work. No matter what religion, what colour skin, what walk of life, what nationality, what culture. If you're a human being you've been gifted with a nervous system that's built for this and it will work. It might not be a flash experience, one that you would write a poem about, but if you meditate regularly, things will change, and you will get experiences that are so beautiful, because you're transcending.

Through the David Lynch Foundation a lot of young people learn to do Transcendental Meditation. From age four or five or six a child could get what they call their walking mantra or their word of wisdom. That's for kids who are old enough to promise and keep their promise that they won't tell their mantra to anyone else. They just have a mantra to say and their teacher will tell them what to do. It's easy and it keeps the stress from sticking to them. And when they're 10, they can get their sitting mantra. And when they're 10 they'll meditate for 10 minutes in the morning and 10 minutes in the afternoon. And as they grow older, they'll add minutes until they work their way up to 20.

You can meditate anywhere. You know, you don't stand on your head. You sit comfortably and close your eyes, and meditate the way you were taught. There's no trying. In fact, trying blocks it. My friend Charlie Lutes, who ran the centre where I started, said the best attitude is, 'Here goes nothing for 20 minutes.' Here goes nothing for 20 minutes and away you go. It's very, very enjoyable and it's always the same, but always different. It's the strangest thing and it's sublime, it's refreshing, it's energising, it brings happiness. It's so incredible that people aren't transcending every day. It's just mind-boggling. Look at the trouble in this world. This brings solutions. This brings happiness, love, energy, creativity, intelligence — it brings it all out for you to enjoy.

BENEFITS AND SIDE-EFFECTS

What you find out is that when you're transcending every day, it's like building up a flak jacket against stress, against depression, against all negativity, against fear, against anxiety, so those things you can look forward to getting less of. The things that used to get you angry or discombobulated, it doesn't happen so easily anymore. As you meditate regularly, you don't really notice the change, but people around you will say, 'Steven, what are you doing? You seem happier. You seem nicer. You don't seem so upset. What is the deal? What is it?' And you realise that you've changed by transcending every day. So it seems sort of normal, but when you think about it, you've gotten happier. The same people that used to stress you, it's like you almost like them!

If you go out and find a drug dealer and get yourself a bag of heroin and shoot that heroin, you would have an instantaneous experience. And for a lot of people it's a very good experience, but they don't own that experience. They had it, but they don't own that. With Transcendental Meditation you're going to unfold that for yourself. There's a lot of side-effects to taking drugs too. There is a side-effect of transcending every day and it's that negativity starts lifting away. It's a win-win situation.

It would be nice to get eight hours' sleep. I mostly get six or seven. Sleep is very, very important and a lot of people have trouble sleeping these days.

You're going to sleep so much better if you're transcending every day. There's no posture necessary. People can sit in a lotus position if they want. They can sit however it's comfortable. I sit comfortably. Then I close my eyes and do it as I was taught. If your body is tired, you will fall asleep in meditation, yes, but it will be more like a nap, and then when you wake up from the sleep you meditate for five or 10 more minutes in that more refreshed state, and then get up and go about your business.

I have never missed a meditation, twice a day, since I started. How did I find time to do that? I don't know. Charlie told me early on, the most important thing you can do for yourself is meditate regularly. To visit the transcendent on a regular basis is big, so when you think about it, it's not that difficult to give it 20 minutes in the morning and 20 minutes in the afternoon. Everybody knows we waste way more than 40 minutes a day anyway, so you might as well put it to good use.

ART AND PLEASURE

I'm what they call an artist and an artist likes to do things on their own. They don't want anybody telling them anything. They don't want to join any club. They want to be on their own, do their own thing, in freedom. So I had a problem with this. I said, 'You mean I'm going to learn a technique that a 10-year-old also does or Sammy who's an accountant or somebody else like this. I'm going to have the same technique. Me, being so special!' So it's something to overcome. The long and the short of it is, it doesn't matter who else is doing it, it's for you. You're the one that gets the technique, and gets the ability to transcend and go as fast as you possibly can to enlightenment. You just have to live your life, but add this to it.

There's no way to tell if Transcendental Meditation has changed my art. I always say, I was creative before I started Transcendental Meditation, but I was not as self-assured. I was not as happy in the doing. I have changed in that I enjoy life more. I enjoy the work more. I like people more. I feel better in my body. I see a bigger, brighter picture. I see, as I say, life becoming more like a game than a torment. I see things that used to stress me, and bring me down and, yes, almost kill me, not having that power anymore over me. They say mankind was not made to suffer. Bliss is our nature. We're supposed to enjoy life and here's a technique that proves that it's possible. You get this technique and stay regular in the practice, you will never be sorry.

KNOW THE DIFFERENCE

I'm not against any of these other types of meditation, but people have to know the difference. Now listen — concentration forms of meditation are basically the same as concentrating on anything — a maths problem, getting something right about a painting. The brain works in the same way with concentration and you have no chance of sinking deeper and transcending. Contemplation, mindfulness, watching your breath, being aware of your surroundings, smelling the roses, being aware of the wind and the leaves in the trees, being aware of nature, feeling it, being with it — it might be relaxing, but you're not going to transcend. You're going to be near the surface still.

It's not mysticism. They might have called it that in the old days, but it's scientific. That's the weird thing. It's as scientific as the wave function of the universe. It's scientific. It's like two plus two is four. You do this technique properly as you were taught, you're going to transcend. And the thing to think about is, Maharishi didn't make this up. This is from the Vedic tradition. It's as old as time itself. It's a way to go within, transcend and unfold your full potential as a human being.

People have all kinds of experiences. Everybody's ball of string unwinds in a different way. So one of the rules in Transcendental Meditation is, 'Take it as it comes.' Do you transcend without the technique? Yes. I'll tell you exactly how it happens. Say you're in a room that's a circle and the walls are white. There are three curtains hanging on the walls: yellow, red and blue. And the three curtains join, so you can't see the white walls anymore. Let's say the yellow is waking state of consciousness, the blue is sleeping state of consciousness and the red is dreaming state of consciousness. Waking, sleeping and dreaming is something that all human beings enjoy. So when you're awake and getting ready to go to sleep, when your head is on the pillow and you're sort of drifting off, you're at the very edge of the yellow curtain, about to go into the blue curtain. And at certain times people get a little bit of that white room in the gap between the curtains and they see white light maybe or they get a feeling, and they say what is that? You transcended, you experienced the white walls, you experienced the transcendental.

One time I was sitting in a chair comfortably, daydreaming and, boom, I see this white light. It was only after I learned Transcendental Meditation that I knew I had transcended. Would I have loved to have that experience again? Yes, but I didn't know how it happened. I didn't know how to do it again. But I got the technique and now I know how. Now I know where the within is. Now I know how to get to the within, because I got Transcendental Meditation. Embrace Transcendental Meditation and you will never be sorry. It is the real thing. It is the whole thing.

~

Chapter 5

The benefits of meditation on body and mind

~

'Suppose you read about a pill you could take once a day to reduce anxiety and increase your contentment. Would you take it? Suppose further that the pill has a great variety of side-effects, all of them good: increased self-esteem, empathy and trust; it even improves memory. Suppose, finally, that the pill is all natural and costs nothing. Now would you take it? The pill exists. It is meditation.'

– JONATHAN HAIDT, Psychologist

Beside the structural and functional modifications that happen in the brain as a result of meditation, I would also like to discuss in this book its benefits on the body's general health. But before jumping for joy let's start with a more sobering critical overview. The fact is that relatively few studies on meditation fulfil all the strict criteria of quality control or are carried out on a large pool of subjects and with proper 'control' conditions. Yet the studies we do have to hand all show that meditation constitutes a powerful form of mental gymnastics that can have positive effects on both the mind and the body. In fact, according to the American Heart Association, meditation can also contribute to lowering the risk of cardio-vascular illnesses.[1] With certain pathologies, meditation can also be used as complementary medicine alongside traditional medicine. Although they do exist, meditation has fewer side-effects and contraindications, but unfortunately its promising potential is still not harnessed in the healthcare sector. The evolution of scientific research on the matter does not enjoy sufficient visibility. This should come as no surprise. Throughout my extensive training, first as a medical doctor and then as a neurologist and end-of-life physician, I was not introduced to meditation or mindfulness in any of the courses. My wife is a psychologist and mindfulness was not part of her training either. However, the education sector is not the only culprit. Industry, and the pharmaceutical industry in particular, has certainly not been in a rush to put meditation on the agenda.

A little less medication, a little more meditation

It was only at the beginning of the 1970s that researchers woke up to the possibilities presented by meditation, and back then pioneers such as Richard Davidson faced scepticism, but even though it is still in its early stages, scientific research on meditation is extremely promising. Over the last 20 years we have seen an important rise in the number of studies being conducted and mindfulness has progressively established itself in medical institutions, thanks to mindfulness-based stress reduction (MBSR) and mindfulness cognitive-based therapy (MBCT).[2] MBSR has played a major role in research on meditation, not only because it is used in many medical centres across Europe and North America, but also because work on it has been standardised, accredited and repeatable, which is crucial for carrying out quality research.

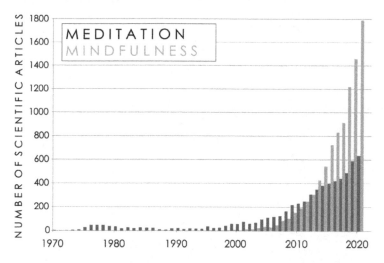

This graph shows the number of scientific articles on meditation (in black) and the number of scientific articles on mindfulness (in grey) over the past 50 years indexed in the National American Medical Library of Medicine (Pubmed Medline) and the US National Institute of Health (NIH). © Steven Laureys (source: www.ncbi.nlm.nih.gov).

Over 1300 clinical studies on meditation and mindfulness have been carried out around the world over the last 20 years.[3] This may sound like a high figure, but it is low compared to, for instance, the 4500 studies on antidepressants carried out each year. Apparently, medication elicits more interest than meditation.

Here are two maps showing the number of controlled clinical studies on mindfulness meditation that have been recorded in different countries since 2000.

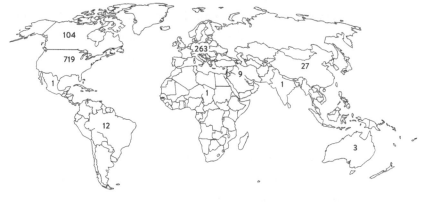

The USA is leading with 719 studies on mindfulness and meditation over the past 20 years. There have been 263 in Europe, and 104 in Canada.

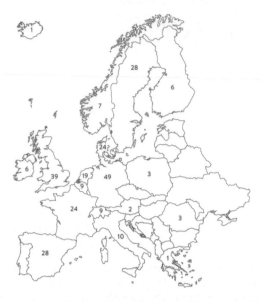

Within Europe, Germany leads with 49 studies on mindfulness and meditation since 2000.

When I take part in international neurology and psychiatry conferences, meditation hardly ever features on the programme. Unfortunately, one has to admit that financial interests and the lure of profit often determine what topics and themes will be reviewed by the medical and scientific community. Studies don't seem to see the light of day without the guarantee of a return on investment and patients' health does not appear to be at the top of the agenda. I am more and more appalled and outraged when I participate in brain disorder conferences. I sometimes have the impression that we, as medics, are at the mercy of the pimps of industry. If we leave things in the hands of the pharmaceutical giants, we are certainly heading towards a future dedicated to Botox and medications that are profitable. When it comes to the treatment of symptoms linked to and exacerbated by stress, the industry simply ignores all alternatives to pills. Only 3 per cent of the 1309 studies on meditation worldwide were financed by industry, compared to 37 per cent of the studies on anti-depressants.

And yet we know perfectly well that meditation can have beneficial effects, even if it doesn't work for all of us or in every case. Indeed, one should refrain from oversimplifying the matter. An analytical study published in the prestigious journal *Nature*[4] unambiguously foregrounded these positive effects: 'Research on meditation carried out over the last two decades confirms overall the view that mindfulness meditation has beneficial effects on mental and physical health as well as on cognitive performance. Recent studies using brain-imaging technology have evidenced the brain areas and networks that are responsible for these benefits. However, the underpinning cell mechanisms remain more obscure. More rigorous studies are needed to understand in greater detail the molecular and neuronal principles at the heart of the changes observed in the brain and that can be linked to mindfulness meditation.'

It appears that we need to carry out more quality studies, that is to say studies that are rigorous in their conceptualisation, execution, analysis, conclusions and publication. Only if we proceed like this can we progress our knowledge in a credible way. And it is crucial that we start to increase the number of clinical studies. We need to work with both a group of meditators and a control group, and the studies need to fulfil strict criteria for excellence. Unfortunately, the studies which are published are not necessarily all clinical studies with adequate control groups. Far from it!

Given that research on meditation is still in its infancy and that the studies are often of questionable quality or the participants involved are too few, it may happen that conclusions contradict each other, which is often the case in scientific research anyway. For instance, one study[5] established that mindfulness meditation was able to ease pain in patients suffering from irritable bowel syndrome, whereas a later analysis of the literature claimed that improvements were relatively insignificant. In many cases we lack solid proof to present irrefutable conclusions and meditation, therefore, often doesn't figure in official medical recommendations. (That being said, doctors themselves have heavily negative biases too!)

In the table overleaf, you can see which medical conditions have been most studied over the last 20 years in relation to mindfulness meditation. You will see that for many studies the results are not yet known or have not been published yet.

Condition	Number of studies	Studies in progress
Psychosis	395	185
Depression	241	97
Anxiety disorder	189	86
Pain	170	75
Quality of life	83	39
Psychological stress	76	31
Overweight	57	23
Cancer	54	29
Skin diseases	54	25
Auto-immune diseases	50	17
Addictions	45	6
Bowel diseases	40	16
Cardiovascular diseases, including hypertension	37	20
Sleep disorders	35	12
Neurocognitive disorders, including dementia	34	24
Diabetes	32	13
Respiratory diseases	32	13
Muscular and joint disorders, including fibromyalgia	31	9
Fatigue (chronic)	30	12
Hormonal disorders	29	14
Multiple sclerosis	15	4
Headaches	15	9
Irritable colon	13	1
Autism	8	7
Tinnitus	5	1

Meditation on prescription

One day, someone asked the Dalai Lama: 'Can meditation be a solution in case of illness?' To which he replied: 'If meditation could cure all health issues, I would not suffer from knee pain any longer.'

To start with, be aware that you don't need to believe everything that's said about meditation and mindfulness. The popular media has a great appetite for health-related fads, and business and marketing specialists are quick to take advantage of people's gullibility. Unsurprisingly, media headlines and social media posts that boast spectacular health benefits are bound to attract the attention of numerous readers and generate lots of Internet clicks. The same goes for meditation – and indeed mindfulness is now slowly starting to generate substantial revenues. In fact, in 2017 the financial value of the mindfulness industry in the USA was estimated at $1.1 billion and it is forecasted to be over $2 billion in 2022. However, one should not forget that meditative traditions did not develop for either medical or financial purposes.

It is high time we carefully evaluate the impact of meditation. When you meditate regularly the structure of your brain changes. Several studies have already evidenced this and we have observed it as well in our studies. But what is the influence of a healthy mind on general health and wellbeing? Don't expect a long list of unrealistic claims. Meditation is no remedy for hair loss. Our approach is first and foremost scientific. We don't rely on personal opinion, but on scientific data. Underpinned by scientific studies we explain what the medical effects of meditation are and which supposed medical effects can be disregarded. We have examined the benefits of meditation on people suffering from chronic pain, anxiety and depression, but meditation is not meant only for the ill or the unhappy. We all struggle with stress from time to time, and there are also interesting connections between mindfulness and creativity, and stimulating attention. Meditation could also contribute not only to improving life, but to lengthening it.

Before examining the results produced by contemplative neuroscience, let us remind ourselves that various neural networks are activated according to the type of meditation that is being practised. Meditation is a global concept or, as my friend psychiatrist and Zen meditation teacher Edel Maex has said, 'Meditation is a box that holds everything you want.' If someone claims that meditation benefits blood circulation, it may be useful to ask yourself what type of meditation would have such benefits? Is it mindfulness meditation, loving kindness meditation, focused attention meditation or transcendental meditation using the repetition of a mantra?

The exact definition, and the standardisation, of meditation and mindfulness are sensitive issues, and one of the challenges of research on meditation, because meditation exercises need to be well defined and reproducible. According to Matthieu Ricard, meditation simply is 'mind training', but everything depends on what you are training for. Training for weightlifting, jogging or badminton are all different things. Likewise, training to develop your attention or training to cultivate loving kindness are different things. The neuronal networks involved will differ and so will the results of the specific training. Each type of meditation has a different neural signature in the brain.

The benefits for health

As a doctor, neurologist and healthcare practitioner, every week I see patients who struggle with headaches, pain, depression, anxiety, burnout, fatigue or sleep disorders. Stress often works as a catalyst. All want to be instantly freed from their suffering and seem to be in search of a miracle cure. 'Doctor, please give me something to get rid of my symptoms!' In the Western world we swallow a huge quantity of pills that inhibit both brain activity and the nervous system. It is clear that medication can be useful, but there are alternatives that aren't magical or pseudo-scientific, such as meditation, mindfulness and other forms of psychotherapy, which may require more effort but which generally have fewer side-effects. Far fewer even! It is worth noting that every day 128 people in the US die from opioid painkiller overdose.[6] An estimated 10 million French people resort to sleeping pills. In Belgium, one third of over-75-year-olds are taking sleeping pills.[7] For many years France and Belgium have been ranked among the biggest consumers of sleeping pills in the world.[8]

The prestigious journal *Nature* has also reported on the theory that meditation may offer interesting treatment potential, asserting in a critical analysis that, 'Mindfulness represents real potential for treating clinical disorders, maintaining a healthy mind and improving wellbeing.' Unfortunately, the quest for alternatives to traditional medicine is littered with traps. There are indeed many false promises floating around and unscrupulous charlatans, even self-proclaimed therapists, who abuse fragile people at a vulnerable point in their life. And that is regrettable! If you are thinking of taking up meditation for a health problem, take advice from a professional specialising in the care that you need – a psychologist, a GP, a neuropsychiatrist or other healthcare practitioner. If you need treatment for a cavity you would go and see a professional dentist, but if you suffer from backache you wouldn't, as you know they wouldn't be able to help you!

You are not defined by your pain

'Pain is inevitable. Suffering is optional.'
AUTHOR UNKNOWN

To the great frustration of health professionals – and particularly patients – pain is the most frequent complaint. When it is chronic, pain often comes hand in hand with depression, apathy, fatigue and insomnia, which in turn can hinder healing. This then becomes a vicious circle. When treating pain, doctors tend to resort solely and too quickly to pills and painkillers. Meditation represents an approach to a healthy lifestyle that also attends more radically to psychological, physical and social needs. As such, it can often prove effective, even if it requires more time and effort, and can be used alongside traditional medication when appropriate.

It is thanks to Dr Jon Kabat-Zinn that mindfulness found a home in medical centres. This professor of molecular biology founded the Mindfulness-Based Stress Reduction (MBSR) Programme. When he was finishing his studies, Jon became interested in yoga and meditation. He then went on a Vipassana retreat, an introspective form of meditation, and had the opportunity try out the famous body scan exercise, which allowed him to discover slowly, carefully and without any preconceived idea, the different sensations of his body. During this exercise he had to stay for hours on the floor in the lotus position and he started to feel intense pain, unlike any he had felt before. And then, during the same body scan exercise, a new perspective on the pain he was feeling gradually imposed itself upon him.

The sensations were still present, but his pain was no longer there. He managed to separate the emotional aspect of pain from the cognitive aspect. This exercise inspired him to take it further: would it not be possible to help patients suffering from chronic pain with meditation? The aim wasn't to heal their pain, but to have them change their perspective on it. This is how the MBSR programme came into being, with the aim not so much of healing patients but enhancing their quality of life.

Does MBSR really work? A team of Dutch researchers decided to review the existing scientific literature.[9] In total, they analysed 22 studies carried out on 1235 chronic pain patients. Their conclusions were moderately positive: in the case of chronic pain MBSR programmes can partially supplement purely medical treatments. Admittedly none of these studies mentioned 'clinical healing', but then painkillers don't heal or cure, and patients were helped in that they suffered less emotionally from the pain. Researchers therefore concluded that meditation, just like other cognitive behavioural therapies, by the way, is at least as effective as medication, although it is important to highlight that mindfulness has fewer side-effects and presents fewer risks of addiction when compared to chemical painkillers.

Meditation doesn't magically cure, but it can alleviate chronic pain and the emotional suffering that comes with it. This is also what clearly came out of my discussion with European decathlete champion Thomas Van der Plaetsen. This high-level athlete had to face being diagnosed with testicular cancer in incredible circumstances. I shall come back to that later, but I can tell you that, thanks to mindfulness, Thomas succeeded in managing the pain he experienced and the emotions that came with being diagnosed and treated for cancer.

A meta-study[10] on seven studies which aimed to identify what mindfulness could bring to cancer patients confirms the impressions that Thomas shared with me: mindfulness interventions have a positive effect on patients' anxiety and depressive symptoms. The study does concede that further studies are needed to determine how lasting the benefits of mindfulness are. Another study,[11] specifically on stress and anxiety experienced during chemotherapy, revealed that mindfulness also had a positive effect on the 57 cancer patients who took part in it.

Pain management and Zen practices
When it comes to the ways in which meditating monks handle pain, some of you will recall the emblematic picture of a Vietnamese Buddhist monk, Tchích Quang Duc, who in 1963 immolated himself, remaining impassive throughout. This example is a sad and extreme one, but it shows the potential power of mental training. If meditation does indeed help alleviate painful sensations, it opens up new hope for patients suffering from persistent pain, such as headaches, arthritis or lower back pain.[12] With this in mind, the Mind & Life institute is supporting a Canadian study on the sensitivity to pain of expert practitioners in meditation.

If you put your hand on a hot plate, two things happen. (Don't try this at home!) First, you burn yourself, which is a physical reaction, and then you shout, 'Ouch', which is an emotional reaction. In a study that involved both expert practitioners in meditation and a control group of non-practising people, a computer-controlled heat source was used to verify whether there was indeed a correlation between meditation and the perception of pain. Experts in Zen meditation managed to dissociate the physical reaction from the emotional one.[13] They perceived the sensation with the same intensity, but felt the pain as something that was less unpleasant.

Pain translates in the brain by the activation of brain areas that are linked to it. What the fMRI tests revealed is that the cortex of the group who did Zen meditation reacted differently to those in the group who did not. My friend the Quebecois psychologist Pierre Rainville described this phenomenon in the following terms: 'Although those who meditated were aware of the pain, the sensation itself was not treated by the brain area responsible for judgment, reasoning and the formulation of memory. We believe that Zen practitioners do indeed feel the sensations, but that they refrain from interpreting or labelling them as being painful.' We don't know yet in detail what mechanisms alleviate pain, but recent studies show that this is not a reaction that involves the brain's opioid receptors.[14]

Insomnia

'Doctor, I have trouble sleeping!' Patients often complain about not being able to fall asleep or about waking up often during the night. It has happened to us all. Once in bed we can't stop worrying about everything that still needs doing or mulling over a colleague's biting comment. We are therefore unable to fall asleep and end up being tired and unproductive. In the long run, lack of sleep can have disastrous consequences on your health. Sleep-deprived patients tend to reach too quickly for sleeping pills, out of despair or because it is easiest. Sleeping pills, however, have rather concerning side-effects in the short and long term. Addiction kicks in very quickly, with the risk that the dose will need increasing over a long period of use. Sleeping pills, just like alcohol, by the way, will induce drowsiness and you fall asleep as you do when given a general anaesthetic – that is to say you fall into a pharmacological coma. But they don't produce a healthy, restorative sleep. Can mindfulness help? A comparative study[15] has evidenced that mindfulness can have a positive impact on sleep without having any side-effects. The mechanisms at stake have not been sufficiently investigated yet and require further studies. One of the theories holds that mindfulness reduces insomnia by better regulating emotions and better controlling the internal voice that holds us awake. The study, however, does not give any details or generally acknowledged instructions based on solid scientific conclusions as to what 'dose' of mindfulness should be recommended to improve sleep.

According to Herbert Benson, the director of the Henry Institute for Mind Body Medicine at the prestigious Massachusetts General Hospital in Boston, one of the best hospitals in the world, it may be that mindfulness – mindfulness being defined as the focus on breathing and the present moment without asking oneself questions about the past and the future – allows us to release a 'relaxation reaction' that will stimulate us into falling asleep. To trigger this process you just have to do the following exercise.

Step 1. Choose a focus that you find relaxing. This can simply be your own breathing or a positive sentence.
Step 2. Let go and relax. Don't think of yourself or what you're feeling. When you feel that your thoughts are straying, breathe in deeply and refocus your thoughts on the object you chose.

Other people will prefer to do the body scan exercise (see page 136) or recite their mantra. Each of us needs to find what works best for him or herself.

Ageing

Does meditation slow down the ageing process? It would seem that Buddha reached the venerable age of 80, which in the 5th century BC represented a rather blessed age in India. Some 2500 years later, scientists have observed that ageing entails the loss of grey matter. We saw that for a 70-year-old, Matthieu Ricard still had a lot of grey matter. Does this mean that meditation could allow us to live longer? Over this last decade, several studies[16] have shown that meditation could potentially protect us against the loss of grey matter. Unfortunately, studies only found a correlation and we can't talk of causality yet, so at this point in time we have too little evidence to answer this question conclusively. However, another avenue may prove more promising: exploring the effect of mindfulness on cell ageing. To better understand this, let us remind ourselves of what telomeres are.

Telomeres are located at the end of your chromosomes and look a bit like the plastic end-pieces you find on your shoelaces. These telomeres shorten over time. This is important, because their length allows scientists to calculate the lifespan of a cell. What is more, telomerase is an enzyme that protects the length of telomeres. High telomerase will therefore have beneficial effects on your longevity. A number of studies dedicated to the relation between telomeres and meditation[17] have revealed that expert meditators have longer telomeres than those who do not meditate. Most of the studies also observe that those who practise mindfulness have increased levels of telomerase. As part of the Shamatha project that I describe later (see page 102), participants did three months of intensive sessions of both mindfulness meditation and loving kindness meditation. Increased telomerase levels were identified in the group who practised meditation. This may seem incredible, but it means that an exercise as simple as sitting down quietly and focusing on your breathing can contribute to your longevity. Despite promising results,[18] identifying the exact conditions in which this process happens, and how long the increased levels last, remains complex.[19]

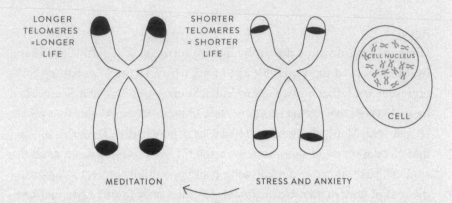

CHROMOSOMES

LONGER TELOMERES =LONGER LIFE

SHORTER TELOMERES = SHORTER LIFE

CELL NUCLEUS

CELL

MEDITATION ← STRESS AND ANXIETY

'I really believe that compassion is crucial to the survival of humanity'

DALAI LAMA

Scientific studies show that meditation as well as other mind-body interventions can be effective in helping us to improve both our physical and mental health. Researchers have recently found an initial plausible explanation for how meditation affects our cells and DNA at a molecular level. It has been shown on several occasions that meditation sessions can influence our chromosomes, the deepest core of our cell nuclei, and in particular the telomeres that form the endings of the chromosomes. When we age, these endings shorten; chronic stress and anxiety seems to accelerate this process. It appears that subjects who meditate a lot enjoy longer telomeres, which offer better cell protection and give a greater chance of longevity. We also have reason to believe that the gene expression (the process by which the instructions in our genes become activated) involved in inflammatory reactions and stress-related illnesses can be positively influenced by meditation. However, substantial research still needs to be carried out in order to shed further light on the mechanisms involved in these specific pathologies. Given that few of the studies fulfil excellence criteria, we do not know the exact role of other healthy lifestyle factors, such as exercise, improved sleep quality or good eating habits. I therefore suggest that you pay more attention to your physical and mental wellbeing by avoiding taking medication unnecessarily. That being said, be aware that meditation does not replace conventional medicine! Combined with physical activity, restorative sleep and healthy eating habits, meditation, as well as other mind-body exercises such as yoga, self-hypnosis and sophrology, but also martial arts such as Tai Chi, can help us have a longer and better life. Compassion meditation may also help you to live a more meaningful life.[20]

Anxiety, stress, depression and inflammation

'Practicing mindfulness considerably improves the regulation of emotions and reduces stress. The fronto-limbic networks involved in these processes show various patterns of engagement by mindfulness meditation.'

YI-YUAN TANG, BRITTA HÖLZEL AND MICHAEL POSNER, *The neuroscience of mindfulness meditation*[21]

Imagine you are a zebra grazing peacefully in the savannah. The weather is beautiful and a light breeze is blowing. Everything is fine. Suddenly you see through the high grass a lion on the lookout. Your amygdala and your emotion network are immediately activated and liberate stress hormones such as cortisol and adrenaline, so that you can save your skin. A few minutes later you are either dead or you are still grazing peacefully as if nothing had happened. The times when we had to flee predators are over. We have now swapped the savannah for a computerised office and a cup of coffee. Unfortunately, mere thoughts, traffic jams, phone calls or stressful emails are now sufficient to trigger a stress reaction similar to the one experienced by the zebra. Yet when pathological stress becomes chronic, illness can be lying around the corner. This mechanism has been amply described by Dr Robert Sapolsky, a colleague neurologist at Stanford, in his book, *Why Zebras Don't Get Ulcers.*[22] There is food for thought in his message. Persistent stress, whether caused by professional, relationship, financial or other circumstances, can slowly kill you, inhibiting the immune system, slowing down growth, and eroding our memory and learning faculties. In order to be less prone to stress and anxiety, one has to learn how to calm down the amygdala and the emotion network. Hence the question, can meditation help with this process?

Although man is not capable of eliminating all sources of stress, he is capable of curbing the devastating effects it has on the body. Thirty minutes of mindfulness meditation or mindfulness stress reduction exercises are sufficient to observe diminished activity in the amygdala,[23] and slowing down the amygdala's activity enables us to have, in turn, a more peaceful mind. This slowing down takes place during meditation, but it has also been observed in the long run, after a sufficient amount of exercises and experience in meditation, in advanced practitioners. Mindfulness therefore allows us to better manage stress that is generated by internal or external causes, not only during meditation but also after. Matthieu Ricard also gave me the following piece of advice in the event that my tendency to mull over problems kicks in: 'If there is a solution, there is no need to worry, and if there is no solution, there is no reason to worry either.'

Working out a reliable research protocol with appropriate control groups is not an easy matter. Let's take the placebo effect, for instance. In most of the rigorous clinical trials, group one receives a treatment whereas group two receives a placebo – fake medication or a pseudo-intervention. Group two believe they are receiving the treatment when in fact they aren't, and the researcher doesn't know who is receiving the real or fake medication either. But how can one create a placebo or 'pseudo-meditation session'? David Creswell, psychologist at Carnegie Mellon, one of the best universities in the United States, has managed, together with his team,[24] to 'falsify' mindfulness sessions. His group was composed of 35 women and men who all suffered from stress caused by long-term unemployment. The first half received authentic training in mindfulness, whereas the second half received relaxation training that didn't take their minds off their worries and stress.

For instance, the teacher in charge of the second group would tell them jokes to entertain them. All participants had a brain MRI taken before and after. They also provided blood samples before the study and four months after. One of the exercises consisted of stretching. The first group had to focus on both pleasant and unpleasant bodily stimuli. The second group, which were doing pseudo-mindfulness, were encouraged to talk during the stretching exercises and ignore their body. After three days of exercise, almost all participants said that they felt alive again and more resistant to the stress caused by unemployment. However, scans performed afterwards showed brain changes appeared almost uniquely in the group who received authentic mindfulness training. In concrete terms, this meant MRI scans showed better communication between the brain areas in charge of treating stress, such as the amygdala, and other areas involved in maintaining and controlling attention, such as the prefrontal cortex. Four months after the experiment blood tests were taken. Although few of them were still doing meditation at that point, only the participants in the authentic mindfulness programme presented with lower levels of interleukin-6, a biochemical marker for the degree of inflammation activation.

This study is particularly interesting because it shows that the health benefits of mindfulness meditation, when compared with a randomised control group intervention, can be explained by objective neurobiological changes that were then analysed by a 'blind' scientist who didn't know who had done the authentic mindfulness exercises, so as to avoid even unconsciously biased results. Other studies have also established that meditation, as it influences genetic expression, can also reduce inflammation.[25]

There is no longer any doubt that we can offer meditation to combat stress and depression. A meta-study carried out at John Hopkins University confirmed this idea.[26] The study analysed 47 quality clinical studies on meditation. In total it covered 3515 participants suffering from various ailments, ranging from depression, anxiety, stress, insomnia and chronic pain. Researchers obtained 'moderate

For depressives, mindfulness can be as effective as an anti-depressant.

proof' that anxiety, depression or pain symptoms were relieved after an eight-week course of mindfulness training, and in particular the Mindfulness-based Stress Reduction programme. And allow me to stress that for depressives, mindfulness can be as effective as an anti-depressant. It would seem that there are too few results available to draw conclusions on mantra-based methods, such as transcendental meditation. However, it is important to highlight that scientists observed no harmful side-effects linked to meditation. This being said, in cases of depression or other illnesses you always need to go and see a healthcare professional before undertaking self-care.

The story of my American colleague, Dr Scott Barry Kaufman

At the start of 2015, Scott Barry Kaufman, who was then 36, had ongoing reservations about meditation, just as I had had a few years before. He held the view that letting one's thoughts wander allowed him to be more creative and he believed that the most committed advocates of mindfulness medita- tion were telling him: 'Stop daydreaming and focus on your breathing.' He had been convinced of the benefits of mind-wandering by his mentor, the Yale psychology professor Jerome Singer, who had undertaken revolutio- nary research on the phenomenon. For Singer, constructive daydreaming constitutes a positive role in our daily life and is indeed beneficial to our creativity. Dr Scott was very dubious about it, but he decided to take part in a mindfulness programme that inflicted upon him a prodigious 40 minutes of meditation per day for eight weeks, i.e. the famous MBSR programme. He had already tried out a number of techniques, ranging from breathing focused meditation to walking meditation through to the body scan. In order to fully dedicate himself to his meditation journey, he also decided to give up Facebook, Twitter, Instagram, Pinterest, WhatsApp and all the other social media platforms that were installed on his computer and smartphone.

There is one small but important additional detail: Dr Scott was prey to spells of deep anxiety and was on the verge of resorting to anti-depressants. Before taking this way out, he decided to grant meditation the benefit of the doubt. After 56 days of meditation, his anxiety was still there, but he had developed a new perspective on the sensations that came with it. He had learnt to be less judgmental about it and to be more compassionate towards himself, towards his emotions and towards others. He understood the extent to which he suffered from the feelings of anxiety he had developed. He also understood that mind-wandering and meditation were not per se in opposition to one another. Interestingly in that respect, a study led by a colleague from Liège[27] showed that daydreaming does not necessarily have detrimental effects on our psychological wellbeing. However, it does affect our tendency to be unaware of the present moment. By contrast, though, when daydreaming becomes persistent mulling over, our wellbeing can be dented.

Give it the attention it deserves!

'Practicing mindfulness improves attention. The anterior cingulate cortex is the region associated with attention and in which changes of activity and/ or of structure in response to mindfulness meditation have most consistently been reported.'

Y I-YUAN TANG, BRITTA HÖLZEL AND MICHAEL POSNER, *The neuroscience of mindfulness meditation*[28]

You may possibly have the impression that meditation is only for people suffering from illness, anxiety or unhappiness. The fact that suffering is indeed a key concept in Buddhism may well serve this belief. As a life-loving Epicurean, I find it hard to welcome such views. Could meditation not be rewarding for happy people too? It is clear that it can be wisely used with patients suffering from specific issues, but people in good health may also want to feel better. We live in an almost constantly oppressive environment. Every day we are overwhelmed with text messages, notifications, emails, newsfeeds and advertisements that we resist with difficulty. Who, among the young and less young, does not honestly check social media before going to sleep? And how long do we wait in the morning to check our emails or go on the Internet? We hardly leave any time for our mind to let go and rest. It would, however, be rewarding for us all to extract ourselves from this constant hyper-stimulation. Our brain is constantly waiting for information, but we apparently have very little awareness of the mental workload it demands.

The American psychologist Herbert Simon describes this phenomenon very aptly: 'Information takes up attention. The abundance of information generates poor quality attention.' When practising meditation you are working on the quality of your attention, but will your attention remain better focused when you don't meditate? And is it possible to prove it scientifically? Let's look at what studies have to say on the matter.

Imagine that you are being shown a whole series of letters. They scroll past your eyes at lightning speed – at ten letters per second. From time to time a number appears between two letters and you are then asked what numbers you saw. If the numbers scrolled past very quickly, it is highly likely that you won't have seen the second one. This phenomenon, called 'inattentional blindness', refers to short absences of attention. In a study carried out by psychologist Richard Davidson[29] this 'inattentional blindness' disappeared in 20 per cent of the people who took an intensive training course in Vipassana meditation, i.e. an introspective form of meditation. You may not find this discovery life-changing, yet scientists had previously considered inattentional blindness as being an immutable given. Professor Davidson and his team demonstrated that experts in meditation are capable of overcoming their inattentional blindness. As a matter of fact, the capacity to identify numbers is not hugely important, but this measurement nevertheless reveals our capacity to identify small changes and therefore to have a better capacity for sustained attention.

Information takes up a lot of attention and the abundance of information often generates poor quality of attention. Our social environment certainly presents an abundance of information. Think of all the subtle, non-verbal signals sent out by our loved ones, our friends or colleagues. If you manage to recognise them you will be better able to understand your environment.

Yuval Harari, best-selling author and discerning mind

The Israeli historian Yuval Harari has written several controversial but very popular books. His first book, *Sapiens*, traced in broad lines the history of humanity. He maintains, in particular, that thanks to our capacity for complex storytelling we have managed to set up complex collaborations that have shaped our society, be it in the form of religion, state organisation or the economy. His book was highly commended and recommended by celebrities such as Barack Obama and Mark Zuckerberg. Writing such a book requires having a discerning mind and it so happens that Harari is a seasoned practitioner of meditation. After his doctorate, he was overwhelmed by questions about the world that he couldn't find any answers to – until on a friend's advice he travelled to India and went on a meditation retreat. He was rather sceptical at first, but after a while Harari started to believe this retreat might well give him some answers.

He now has been meditating twice a day for 17 years and every year he goes on a two-month retreat where he does silent Vipassana meditation. 'Meditation has helped me to flourish in my career,' he has said. Without it, he would have continued to write about medieval military history rather than about the history of humanity. Focus and attention are among the aptitudes he succeeded in developing thanks to meditation.

According to Harari, training your mind to focus on something like breathing allows you to focus your attention on things much broader than the mere counting of breaths you take. It is a mental exercise that allows you to have an enhanced capacity for concentration in everyday life. But things are not that simple. When he started, he could only focus his attention for a few seconds. Later on, meditation allowed him to discriminate between fiction and reality, between what pertains to the real world and what pertains to narrative and is a fabrication of the mind.

Yuval Harari believes that these silent retreats are particularly stimulating. During his stays in meditation villages, there is nothing to distract him: no television, no emails, no telephone and no books. He writes without saying anything. There is only the present moment when he focuses on what happens and the earthy reality of it. He is then able to see things about himself he does not like or phenomena in the world that he does not like either; things that, in another context, he would otherwise have ignored or brushed aside. During these retreats, Harari always starts with basic bodily observations: 'I start with inhaling and exhaling, with observing my belly and my legs, and once I have connected with these parts of my body I can observe everything that happens. Everything becomes clearer in my mind and I can understand what is happening in there. It is difficult to take stock of anger, anxiety or boredom if you are not able to observe your breathing.' As he progresses in his retreat, his mind becomes more focused and perceptive. He does not do anything if he feels he is overwhelmed by anger; neither does he brush his anger away or attempt to fight it off. Only neutral observation matters to him then. After a certain time, he is able to identify the causes of his anger and his anxiety. In our daily lives, it often happens that we feel anger, anxiety or boredom, but it is rare that we take the time to observe it.

What do we really feel when we are angry? Like Yuval Harari, I believe that the manifestations of such emotions are among the most surprising things I have had the opportunity to observe. I hope you will have a similar experience on your personal journey towards meditation.

Creative minds
According to film director David Lynch, only meditation allows him to take the plunge and catch what he calls 'big fish', that is the ideas he uses as ingredients for his films and music. There are many other creative minds who practise or used to practise meditation, including celebrities such as Yoko Ono, Leonard Cohen, Richard Gere, Moby, and Jack Kerouac. And, as I mentioned above, Yuval Harari is also a wholehearted Vipassana meditation enthusiast who links the quality and content of his work to his practice of meditation. These are not just words. Studies have shown that a well-developed capacity for observation is a reliable precursor for creativity.[30] What's more, this capacity is

reinforced by open awareness meditation and improves not only our working memory, but also our cognitive flexibility, which are all essential ingredients in the creative process.

An interesting meta-analysis[31] looked into how creativity and mindfulness are related, and carefully reviewed 20 articles on the topic. The question remains as to how we measure creativity. Scientists have identified the capacity 'to think differently' as one of its crucial aspects. A person who is easily able to think differently will be able to formulate a greater number of new ideas. Often this greater number of new ideas will produce more creative solutions. Scientists have concluded that people who do mindfulness seem to have more ideas than people who don't.

Empathy and compassion need cultivating!

When we have the impression that someone is trying to deceive us, we have the tendency to respond violently. We become angry and demand that justice be done. Sometimes we go as far as requesting that the 'bad people', the originators of this unfair behaviour, be heavily punished. We give the impression that that matters more than compensating the victims. Imagine that you have been witness to a theft in broad daylight. Two youngsters rip the handbag from an old lady and flee on a scooter. This spectacle shakes you to your core to the extent that you would like to see these youngsters perish in a dungeon. These thoughts of vengeance may prevail over a certain compassion towards the old lady in question. Social norms in place will, in the first instance, define the gravity of the sentence that will be imposed on the offender. In our day and age, and in our part of the world, one does not cut off the hands of thieves any longer, contrary to what was the custom a few hundred years ago. Then our social preferences play a decisive role. The fact that an unfair act makes you angry will, for instance, determine to a large extent the severity of the sanction you would like to see imposed on the perpetrators. In other words, your state of mind will for a large part determine your propensity towards leniency or your need for revenge. The question, therefore, is to know whether meditation can influence your social preferences.

A study carried out at the Max Planck Institute for Neurosciences in Leipzig looked into the effects of mental training, such as loving compassion meditation, on our tendency to punish offenders or compensate victims. During this study a group of experts in meditation and a group of participants who had no experience in meditation were asked to play several versions of the 'dictator game'. The scientists recruited a group of meditation superstars, who on average all had more than 40,000 hours of mental training under their belt. Among them was also Matthieu Ricard, the very person who inspired this book. Several people who had never done any meditation were selected to constitute the control group. The experts in meditation also had experience in compassion meditation.[32] Participants played different versions of the game. Besides the usual fee paid for participating in experiments, all participants were given an additional fee, which varied according to the decisions taken during the game. They had the option to sanction the dictator financially, either as direct victims of the mean dictator or as witnesses to the treatment inflicted by the narrator on another anonymous player. Results were quite conclusive. Compared to the control group, Matthieu and his expert colleagues, as victims of injustices, had a lesser tendency to punish the dictator. Those who did not meditate indicated that they felt greater anger when faced with injustice.

Our social preferences are not set in stone, but can evolve.

The data thus suggests that those who practised meditation felt less anger when they were the victim of unfair treatment and therefore sanctioned such behaviour less severely. However, when it came to sanctioning injustices inflicted on others, those who meditated chose punishments just as severe as those imposed by the control group made up of those who did not meditate. Participants also played a round in which they had to compensate victims. The results showed that those who meditated would pay out compensation more often. The study showcased how justice is perceived differently, with the group of those who meditated being less receptive to the gratifying aspects of revenge. These differences suggest that our social preferences are not set in stone, but can evolve, and that altruistic reactions, when confronted with injustice, can be shaped by mentally cultivating motivation, altruism and compassion.

TESTIMONIAL: THE SHAMATHA PROJECT

Participants reported that they felt their wellbeing had improved and their existence was more meaningful.

~

In 2007 Cliff Saron, a neuroscientist from the University of California, led a study carried out in Boulder, Colorado, on the effects of meditation.[33] So what happened in Boulder? Sixty participants were cherry-picked and divided into two groups. The first group of 30 people went on a retreat to do meditation exercises for six to 10 hours a day. They also had to take all sorts of tests. The other 30 participants constituted the control group, which had to take exactly the same tests, at the same time, without doing the intensive meditation exercises programme. As soon as the first group was finished, the control group followed the exact same meditation programme. This thorough approach allowed scientists to see if they obtained similar results for the two groups over their period of meditation.

The project concluded that, in terms of being able to focus, the participants of both groups were able to better distinguish between lines that had negligible colour differences. This improvement could still be observed up to five months after the retreat in the participants. In terms of emotions and wellbeing, the participants' psychological wellbeing improved considerably. Even five months after the training programme, the participants reported that they felt their wellbeing had improved and their existence was more meaningful. Participants were also asked to watch violent film scenes and were themselves filmed for the occasion. Both the authors and victims of violence appeared on the screen. Researchers deduced from participants' facial expressions that the group who had taken the meditation programme first showed less aversion and was more emotionally engaged than the control group.

~

Chapter 6

Do what you can!

~

'In theory there is no difference between theory and practice. In practice, there is.'
— YOGI BERRA, Baseball player, 1925–2015

A disciple asks a Zen master: 'How long does it take to be able to experience Awakening?' 'Maybe 20 years,' answers the master. 'And if I am in a hurry?' asks the disciple again. 'In that case, it is 50 years,' concludes the master.

No scientist should passively accept as being the absolute truth what is written in a book or what their teachers tell them. It is this critical attitude that allows him to reject the accepted truth of the present day and create the (transitory) truth for the future. I believe that I have such a rebel streak in me and indeed I never excelled at abiding by arbitrary rules. Let me give you an example. When I was attending my first yoga classes, during the difficult time in my life, my yoga teacher used to tell me off. For instance, I had once smoked just before and after a session focusing on breathing exercises and smelt of cigarettes. When my teacher compassionately explained to me how silly that was, I said to myself, 'She is right. I will do what I can.'

This is precisely the reaction I hope to trigger in you now. When I browse through other books on meditation, I find the slightly condescending tone adopted by some authors who try to encourage their readers to do a certain number of meditation exercises per day always somewhat disturbing. But don't get me wrong. If you manage to stick to your two daily meditation sessions and make that a routine, I can only applaud and encourage you to persist.

The more you practise regularly and frequently, the greater the benefits of meditation are. But I prefer to remain realistic and avoid imposing fixed exercises, whatever they are. When I see patients who suffer from neurological problems, such as chronic pain or insomnia, I encourage them, alongside the traditional medication they are prescribed, if needed, to take up a better lifestyle: a better quality of sleep, mental and physical activity, including psychological support and meditation exercises. When patients come back for a follow-up appointment and show that they have done all they could, it makes me really happy.

We all may experience situations or go through periods that do not allow us to find either the time or courage to dedicate ourselves knowingly to formal meditation on a daily basis and at a precise moment of the day. We are human beings made of flesh and bone; we work and have a family life; we have professional obligations as well as time off for leisure. And if I am perfectly honest, I would say that meditation need not be onerous but rather a means to take a step back at moments that suit us and when we most need it; that is, when illness, pressure and the chaos of daily life and thoughts take their toll. The reality is that even repeated short training is enough to produce significant change. What matters is regularity rather than untimely effort, just as is the case for physical exercise. Changing your attitude and acknowledging the benefits of sport and fresh air are not enough to reap these benefits: you actually have to train and practise. There is no shortcut, despite what self-help manuals might say. What meditation boils down to is a small moment of quiet and control that you offer to yourself as a gift. If, however, you have the impression that meditation is just part of a long list of numerous existing obligations, I believe you will be likely to lose out on all it has to give.

Of course, it would make no sense to believe that we will all become Buddhist monks like Matthieu Ricard. In fact, I like to tease him from time to time, telling him that if we all became monks the world would stop spinning. If we spent all our life meditating, we would never achieve things, such as developing new treatments or new technologies. The comparison may be extreme, I grant you, but what matters here is that everyone needs to finds the balance that is right for them, the way it works best for them, and integrate meditation into their lives as they see fit, in order to reap all its benefits. When you start, don't aim too high. And don't be too harsh on yourself.

It's a bit like doing physical exercise. Let's say you like running. If one day you are training with a marathon runner you will immediately come to realise that he has better endurance and stamina than you. So what? That should not prevent you from enjoying your short Sunday morning jog.

I do what I can when I can
And no one should be allowed to tell you that running less than 5 kilometres and at a speed less than 10 kilometres per hour is ridiculous. In 2019 I ran the New York marathon with my eldest son Hugo. We didn't achieve an extraordinary time, but made it to the finishing line and enjoyed the full run. I was happy with what we achieved and really proud of it!

That's why I would encourage you to regularly take a step back in order to observe yourself, your behaviour, your emotions and the pace of your lifestyle before returning to your cruising speed. I would also encourage you to take moments of rest when you need them. I am probably less demanding than Matthieu, who insists that you should practise every day, again and again, just as if you were learning to play the piano. As for me, I am more easy-going, I do what I like – what I can and when I can.

I can only urge you to try and delve into this state of consciousness, mental exercise, and calm on a daily basis, but what I don't want, though, is to force everyone to meditate every day at a set time and for a set period of time in the lotus position. If you do your best and have the will to live your life more mindfully, the rest will follow. Once you have learned some basic techniques you can be mindful and meditate informally throughout your day: at work, while commuting, in the shower or when you take a stroll, cook or put on your make-up.

The impression that meditation is part of an imposed routine for which you don't really have time may hinder its practice. Before we go into the details of different techniques of formal or informal meditation, I would like to answer some questions you may have as a beginner.

Where should I meditate?

The answer is: wherever you like. A session of formal meditation is easier to do in a quiet and secluded place where you won't be disturbed by anyone. but in principle you can practise meditation everywhere – in the train or on the bus, in the office or even when you are running. For informal meditation, you can just choose a place where you feel comfortable at that very moment. After a little of training, you will even be able to engage in it during difficult moments, whether you are on an airplane, in a line at the grocery store, in a traffic jam, or at the office before or after a stressful meeting.

What position should I adopt to meditate?

Choose the position that is the most comfortable to you. For many, being seated crossed-legged, back comfortably straight, eyes closed, is the ideal position, but you can also just sit on a chair. Or you may prefer to sit on a bench, to lie down or to remain standing. For me, that works well too.

What matters most is that you feel comfortable while being attentive. What came out of my conversations with Matthieu, and he insists on this matter in his books too, is that posture affects our mental state. He teaches that slouching induces a fuzzy, tense and agitated mind.[1]

How long should I meditate for?

As long as you like. Often experts in meditation such as Matthieu suggest that you start with five or 10 minutes, and that you progressively lengthen the sessions up to about 20 minutes if you want to see lasting changes kick in. But in principle each minute, even each second, is beneficial, as studies have proven.[2] For children a few minutes are enough to start with. Even if your session just consists of taking a few deep breaths or pausing to observe why you have reacted in a certain way in a specific situation, you are benefiting from a precious moment of full awareness, of quiet and relaxation. Do what you can for as long as you can. No more and no less.

When should I meditate?

At a moment when you need it or have the time for it. Ideally, it is good idea to set up a routine time, for instance when you wake up. After a while it will become part of your healthy lifestyle, like brushing your teeth. But then again, do what you can. If it suits you best, start the day with a short session, but it may well be that on another day a good meditation exercise before going to sleep is exactly what you need. Or before an important meeting, so that you can relax before going in. Or else, if your partner, boss or kids haven't stopped complaining, you can grant yourself a little moment just to yourself. The ideal moment for meditation is the one that suits your own needs.

With whom should I meditate?

With all those you would like to be with. For some, meditating with a timer is enough; for others, there is nothing like a class and meditation in a group. For others, it might involve using an app or one of the many guided sessions you can find on YouTube. I am fascinated by new technologies, so I tried out several meditation apps. And I shall come back to this in one of the following chapters.

Some people start meditating when they feel anxious or depressed. When you don't feel good about yourself, you have a greater tendency to depend on others. I therefore would recommend that you don't throw yourself into the hands of just any teacher or non-qualified guru.

Unfortunately, there are some charlatans and self-proclaimed therapists out there. If you want to learn meditation or mindfulness as a patient, discuss it with your treating physician and choose a teacher who has received qualified training. But then again, this quest should remain a personal one. Yet even if you were taught by the Dalai Lama, Tsoknyi Rinpoche or Lama Zeupa, to mention just three great masters whom I have had the pleasure of meeting, or even any other meditation master, it wouldn't mean that success is guaranteed! When I take up the topic of meditation with my patients, some will go and purchase books by the psychiatrist Christophe André[3] or the philosopher Frédéric Lenoir.[4] That can be great start and many have already found valuable help this way.

I am sure that you understand what I mean: when you try out the exercises and tools I offer in this book, you will be able to use them in your own fashion, at your own level and your own rhythm. Some teachers and books will maintain that you need to meditate for at least 40 minutes a day in order to reap benefits, but let me reassure you, I won't impose anything. Rather, I hold the view that meditation is like riding a bike: you somehow never forget. No doubt Matthieu would cut in, pointing out that this is only true if you have already acquired good expertise! I hope no one forgets how easy it is to ride a bike, even when it has been safely locked away in your shed. Maybe we all have the skill for mindfulness in us as children and just need to reconnect to the mental power we once enjoyed as youngsters.

During the rough patch I went through, I always found my yoga teacher's precious advice very helpful. In particular, she would repeat with endless patience: 'Do what you can!' To classify yoga techniques according to whether they are good or bad doesn't make sense. Lama Zeupa, with whom I did a meditation retreat, was of the same opinion. You may lie on a mat meditating for hours, but you may also inhale and exhale mindfully throughout the day and feel an enormous difference.

TESTIMONIAL: JOACHIM MEIRE

**'If you are able to spend hours on your smartphone,
surely you can find five minutes to meditate.'**

~

*When one evokes meditation, many people spontaneously think of yoga. That
should come as no surprise since yoga and meditation have much in common.
My colleague Joachim Meire, a nurse, yoga teacher and experienced meditator,
tells us here about his own personal journey and explains the link that exists
between the two practices.*[5]

PROTRACTED HOLIDAYS AND FREE DIVING

At the end of my nursing studies, I felt like going on holiday for just a week.
I took a flight to Egypt and stayed three months. I was swept away by the
splendours of the undersea world and became a diving instructor. At some
point I was taking out a group of parachutists. Each day we would go out on
the boat for the evening outing. In this group there was a lady who told me
about breathing techniques, such as pranayama or yoga, which helped her
clear her mind and slow down her metabolism. I found it fascinating and went
for it! A new world opened up to me. For the first time my mind was totally at
peace, a bit like turbulent waters that then calm down. I also do free diving,
which means that I don't use oxygen cylinders. Breathing techniques help
me to stay underwater for longer.

YOGA AND MEDITATION

Once back home I happened upon a brochure advertising yoga classes.
It offered vinyasa sessions, which is an intensive form of yoga, different
from the meditative yoga that the lady in Egypt had told me about. I know
much more about yoga and meditation now. I have learnt to be more
disciplined and less impulsive. In the past I would tend to do things at
the drop of a hat and then leave them unfinished. Meditation and yoga
positions (asanas) have taught me how to focus on possibilities rather
than limits.

I am a sportsperson, and love surfing and yoga. Because I have arthritis, I can't carry out all my ambitions, but I am grateful for all I can still do. Yoga is for almost everyone. It is one of the few physical activities that can be done at all ages. It is commonly thought that you need to be flexible to do yoga, but it is precisely those who are as stiff as a board who will benefit from taking up yoga. Yoga offers benefits to both body and mind. That is one of the reasons why athletes of different disciplines make it part of their overall training programmes. It enhances concentration and rids the body of tensions. In the Western world, many people accumulate tensions sub-consciously, often in the region of the shoulders, neck and lower back. The fact that we are always bending our heads towards our smartphone or our computer make this postural imbalance worse. Our unconscious anxieties also play tricks on us and we are not able to enjoy the present moment. The very core of yoga helps to remedy these ills.

I am currently offering training, and meditation forms an important part of my classes. In order to meditate, you need to be able to stay still for at least 10 minutes. For many, this is a real challenge. During yoga sessions, you need to adopt positions that force you to find your physical balance, which in the long run also helps you to remain still more easily. That is why yoga is a good supplement to meditation – at least if you do the positions correctly. Many people take up yoga because they are attracted to its physical aspect. They will come through my studio door saying, 'I don't like meditation so much, but I would like to take care of my body.' But after a while, they often want to venture into meditation. For me, it is the opposite. I always start my class with a fine-tuning exercise, when I prepare the mind for a yoga state, and I finish with a meditation exercise. I teach my students several Kelee techniques. These rather simple methods are very popular with surfers and they allow you to focus your attention on the top of your skull and then progressively take it down the body.

Over time, yoga and meditation techniques become richer and richer, by dint of the repetition. I always start my day with a yoga session and end it with meditation. When I skip this routine for a few days I notice that I become more irritable, that I start to brood and that I find it difficult to let go. Some people will take 10 sessions of meditation and think, 'That's it. I am all set!' It doesn't work that way. Endurance demands discipline. All those who are capable of it manage to keep up their concentration over the long run. I often tell my students, 'If you are able to spend hours on your smartphone, surely you can find five minutes to meditate.' It is far better to take five minutes on a daily basis to create silence around you than to meditate for an hour once a week. It's just like when you learn a foreign language. Everybody is able to learn Russian if they take lessons and practise regularly.

MEDITATION ON A SURF BOARD

I love yoga, but I also love surfing, which is another of my passions. And my surf board has much in common with my meditation mat. When one surfs one is faced with one's anxieties, doubts and inner demons. One plays with nature and its elements. Waves have travelled thousands of kilometres and their power is impressive. Each wave is different. You therefore need to remain master of each moment and keep focusing on your breathing. These are the elements one also finds when one gazes into one's inner world.

~

Chapter 7

It all starts with breathing

~

'Feelings come and go like clouds in a windy sky.
Conscious breathing is my anchor.'

– THICH NHAT HANH, Peace activist and Buddhist monk

Come to think of it, I know almost nothing about you. I have no clue why you are reading this book or where you are, whether you are sitting, lying or just standing. Neither have I got any idea about what you might be thinking of the book. I don't even know your name, whether you are a woman or man, young or old, single or married. But what I know for sure is that you breathe and that you are breathing now. As you read these lines you are breathing, sometimes consciously, but most of the time unconsciously. Most of the time breathing is taken for granted, but it is one of the most remarkable phenomena. First of all, breathing allows us to be alive. What is more, breathing also entails all sorts of reactions in our brain. That is precisely why if you have a heated discussion or a difficult meeting it is wise to inhale and exhale calmly, in a controlled way.

Breathing mindfully

Breathing is one the most powerful functions of the body. It is also one of the automatic vital functions that you can consciously control, which, by contrast, is impossible when it comes to blood circulation or digestion. Clearly, most of the time you breathe without noticing you're doing it and have as little control over the process as you do when your stomach digests food.

By the way, this is also the case when you are sleeping. If we didn't have the capacity to breathe automatically and unconsciously it would be very difficult for us to focus both on breathing and on our work, to do the cleaning and think about driving our kids to school. However, the fact that it is in our power to choose at any given time to breathe in a conscious and controlled manner constitutes an enormous asset. For instance, we can breathe more slowly and more profoundly by either engaging our chest or belly. We can hold our breath or breathe out fully by expelling all the air from our lungs. You can breathe through your nose or through your mouth, in a regular, rapid or jagged fashion. But given that we breathe all day long, we often forget to what degree this conscious and unconscious breathing is peculiar. That is a pity, of course, because our capacity to control our breathing and to breathe consciously is very beneficial to the brain. That's why I like

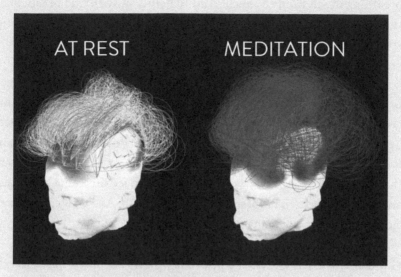

© Steven Laureys, with the participation of Rajanikant Panda, an engineering PhD student in our research team who also practises meditation, and our colleague Dr Srivas Chennu from the University of Kent. (This type of analysis has been published in the journal *Brain*.[1])

'Your life is shaped by what you focus on'
TONY ROBBINS, SELF-TAUGHT LIFE COACH

The pictures above represent the EEG measurement of the electrical activity taking place in Matthieu Ricard's brain (see page 31) during a state of normal consciousness, when thoughts come and go, as well as during 'focused attention' meditation, with the focus on his breathing.

The brain's electric activity and the alpha[2] waves' connectivity increase considerably when Matthieu focuses his attention on his breathing. The image shows the intensity of the brain connections. The blacker the lines, the more intense the communications between the regions of the brain. As you can see, meditation does not consist of 'thinking of nothing'; neither does it inhibit brain activity — on the contrary. The same observations can be made during other types of activities, such as viewing an artwork, listening to a piece of music or being in a state of 'flow' when playing sport. The study we carried out with Guillaume Néry, a high-performance athlete and world champion in free diving, allowed us to obtain similar images when he was focusing on his breathing. Scientific studies have further evidenced that you don't necessarily need to be either an expert in meditation like Matthieu Ricard or a high-performance athlete like Guillaume Néry. During meditation each of us can feel this type of mental wellbeing and those benefits in our brains. Doing the exercises and perseverance are crucial. Practice improves performance!

breathing meditation so much. And to help you with this practice, in this chapter I will be suggesting a number of exercises and offering specific breathing tips.

Breathing meditation has been one of the most popular meditation practices for a very long time. In particular, oriental medicine has used it for centuries and I am also trying to incorporate it into my medical practice. Yet beware – just because it's an ancient practice doesn't mean that it's in itself true and effective! Controlled breathing brings much more to the body than just oxygen. Research has shown that controlled breathing has visible and tangible effects on the brain's activity and health. And Guillaume Nery's story bears testimony to that.

Guillaume Néry is a French world-champion free diver. My research team has had the opportunity to study his brain. Free diving is one of the deep-sea diving disciplines that is done without oxygen cylinders. Free divers hold their breath throughout the whole diving exercise. My friend Guillaume, whose last world record dates back to 2015, went down as deep as 139 metres and he actually lost consciousness. As we studied his brain, we made a fascinating discovery. Strangely enough, it appears that his brain has a striking resemblance to the brain of great meditation experts.

First, we were able to observe that free diving and his breath control training had not damaged his white or grey matter. Our study took an even more fascinating turn when we started to measure his brain activity while he was holding his breath. He held his breath for seven minutes and 50 seconds in the fMRI and seven minutes and 15 seconds connected to the 256 electrodes of the EEG. To our great surprise, the lack of oxygen did not slow down his brain activity. On the contrary, we noticed that some brain networks recorded more intense activity. Just as with the great meditation experts, the brain networks activated by inner perception, consciousness and attention were the most active. In contrast, the communication between the brain areas responsible for motor activity and verbal communication, as well as the general activity level in these areas, decreased. This means that when Guillaume is free diving he experiences the same stable states of peacefulness, concentration and wellbeing than all the great masters experience when they meditate, while, like them, remaining fully conscious and alert.[3]

When we breathe, the body absorbs oxygen and rejects carbon dioxide, but you probably want to know what will happen in your brain if you do a breathing meditation exercise. The answer is simple: every time you slowly exhale your heart beats a bit slower and your stress levels go down.

Let's try it. Breathe in deeply through your nose, counting to four. Making sure your stomach is inflated and your chest is filled with air. Hold your breath for the count of four and then, again on the count of four, gently breathe out all the air held in your lungs.

Do you notice how relaxed you feel? This feeling of relaxation can be easily explained and, although we will use to a few basic neurology concepts, rest assured you will soon understand what I mean.

The part of our nervous system that you cannot control is called the autonomic nervous system. This system has two main branches: the sympathetic nervous system (comparable to a gas pedal and bringing excitement such as when you are under stress and preparing for action in front of potential danger) and the parasympathetic nervous system (comparable to a brake pedal and bringing relaxation and calm when you feel secure). These two systems regulate the body's vital functions. They work continuously and both control opposite actions. Their functioning can also be influenced by physical and mental stimuli.

When I say that the sympathetic and parasympathetic nervous systems control opposite actions, I mean that they have opposite functions. The sympathetic nervous system corresponds to our 'fight or flight' system and our parasympathetic nervous system corresponds to our 'rest and digest' system.

The first prepares the body to face up to a stressful situation – to fight or flee. The heart rate shoots up, your blood pressure and sugar levels increase, and your pupils dilate. It constitutes a natural stress mechanism for survival. Yet when the sympathetic nervous system is constantly stimulated by ongoing chronic stress, the pressure and sustained vigilance take their toll and become harmful to the body and mind.

As for the parasympathetic nervous system, it has an appeasing influence and a dampening effect. It slows down the heart rate, and encourages digestion and the absorption of nutrients into the organism. One of the main components of this system is the vagus nerve. It owes its name to the fact that it covers such a vast territory of the body (*vagus* means wandering in Latin), as it starts in your brainstem, goes down the neck and then innervates the whole upper body, thus ensuring that brain signals are adequately transmitted to the body. It links the brain to the tongue, pharynx, vocal cords, lungs, heart, stomach, intestines and the various glands producing hormones that influence our digestion and metabolism. What is of utmost relevance here is the connection and interaction between brain, lungs and heart, as they are all organs in charge of crucial vital functions.

So why am I telling you all this? Because controlling the parasympathetic nervous system and the vagus nerve is key to controlling thoughts, emotions, and stress levels. But didn't I start out by saying that we could not control these nervous systems? That is indeed the case. Normally you can't control the autonomic nervous system, but this is the exception that proves the rule. If you breathe in calmly and hold your breath for a while before exhaling slowly, you will stimulate your vagus nerve, which in turn will have a soothing effect on your body and brain. That is why training in meditation breathing is a formidable tool for controlling and consciously inhibiting unconscious stress reactions. As such, it allows us to modify our brain activity (as we have demonstrated in our lab[4]) to overcome anxiety, to lower blood pressure and sugar levels (and thus reduce the risk of cardiovascular diseases), to strengthen the immune and metabolic systems, and to have a positive influence on numerous pathologies. Doing meditation does not mean, however, that you may stop your traditional medical treatments, but it can benefit our concentration capacity[5] and the many symptoms related, caused or worsened by chronic stress.

Now back to work!

That was the theory, now let's get back to practical matters. Of course, I don't expect you to take up formal meditation as soon as you close this book. The exercises, the techniques and the tips that are given here are to be used as tools and guidance. You can apply them when and where you wish. And, as you now know, you can adapt them and shape them to your own liking. I'll set out a general introduction to breathing meditation. Then I'll give you a few tips to help you practise it. Last but not least, I'll explain a number of specific breathing techniques that you may want to implement during your meditation sessions, if you feel like it.

Choose a place where you would like to meditate and, whether you choose to sit, stand or lie down, make yourself comfortable. I personally prefer to sit crossed-legged on a small cushion, but please feel free to choose the position that suits you best. What matters is that you are comfortable while keeping alert. Your position should not bring about any physical discomfort, but it should not induce immediate drowsiness, unless of course you do the exercise with the intention of falling asleep.

Simply start by consciously observing your breathing. At this stage you should not yet apply any specific breathing technique. The main objective is to remain conscious and alive to every breath, to relax and to rid yourself of the tension in your body progressively, with each breath you take. This way you will be able to open up and have a more relaxed attitude, even if, to start with, it feels odd to be sitting, standing or lying there. You will get used to it. Don't be judgemental about yourself. Continue to breathe calmly and focus on your breathing, and your mind and body will automatically unwind.

The chances are that within seconds you will be distracted by your own thoughts and feelings, as well as the noises around you... Don't be too disappointed and accept the fact for what it is, without asking yourself too many questions. And don't dwell on it! Observe your 'monkey mind', the way your thoughts and perceptions wander all over the place. That is the essence of the meditative state: to be able to recognise that a number of things are happening without minding them too much, merely accepting them. You will observe that those thoughts don't linger; that they come and go spontaneously. What then remains is just you and the object that you want to focus on, in this case your breathing.

As soon as you have relaxed into your chosen position, maintain your attention on breathing for a few minutes. At the start, don't force anything by trying to implement a certain number of specific breathing techniques. Inhale and exhale, and let yourself be carried away by all the sensations you experience. I would invite you to focus on the sensation of the air that tickles your nostrils, and then on the movement of your belly and chest when you inhale and exhale. Discover what your breathing does to your body. The objective is to remain focused on your breathing without necessarily controlling it. Try to really enjoy the simple fact that you are breathing. Breathing can prove very relaxing, soft, soothing and restorative. The more you learn how to enjoy it, the easier it will be for you to maintain your attention on breathing.

What can help you refocus your attention when thoughts go wandering off is to count during your breathing, up to ten: 1, 2, 3... Or to name the breathing movements: inhale, exhale, inhale, exhale. You can also visualise the air that goes in and out of your lungs. Take the time to enjoy this moment when concentrating on your breathing is the only thing that matters. This will help you keep your focus. Set aside your shopping lists, deadlines and timetables... The only thing that matters now is to inhale and exhale. And if your shopping list comes back to haunt you, don't worry, because thoughts come and go, and that is normal. Just refocus on your breath. Again and again and again.

The chances are that to start with your thoughts will wander quite a lot or that you will be distracted by the smallest sensory stimulus. Don't beat yourself up over it. And don't be too harsh on yourself. A wandering mind is only natural. You have always left your brain to its own devices. As a consequence, it is no surprise that it doesn't immediately do what you ask it to. This doesn't mean, however, that you are not meditating correctly. These thoughts and distractions are just like clouds that go through your mind. Don't try and analyse them, and don't be too critical of yourself. On the contrary, it is a good thing you noticed that you were distracted. Accept that your thoughts have wandered and refocus again on your breathing and the benefits you feel. The fact that you become aware of your thoughts wandering will be addressed in the next chapter, which focuses on mindfulness meditation.

Continue doing your breathing exercises, focusing your attention on your breathing and taking stock of the fact your thoughts are wandering, so that you can refocus on your breathing until the end of the meditation session.

You will determine the length of the exercises yourself, by setting a timer for two, five or 10 minutes, for instance. I would suggest that once you've finished you remain seated for a little while, so that you can enjoy the lingering sensations. Then open your eyes wide, stretch, stand up carefully and continue your day with a new perspective on it.

In order to keep your attention focused on breathing, the following tips will come in handy. Think of them as a First Aid kit for meditation.

- Count all the full breaths you are taking (1, 2, 3...).
- Name the phases of your breathing (inhale, exhale, inhale, exhale).
- Repeat a brief phrase continuously (just breathe, just breathe).
- Feel your breathing. Put your hands on your belly or chest and focus on the movement caused by your breathing.
- Visualise your breathing. You may, for instance, imagine that your breathing is like a swing. With each inhalation you swing backwards with each expiration you swing forwards. You can also visualise your breathing as a sea wave that moves up the sand when you inhale and that falls back when you exhale.
- You can also use any evenly beaded necklace to trace your breathing. Like using prayer beads, it is only a matter of fingering one bead forward for each breath you take. This technique allows your breathing to become more tangible and you will no doubt find it easier to focus your attention.
- Set a timer to control the length of your meditation session. This will allow you not to worry about that during meditation and instead focus entirely on your breathing.

- Start with just a few minutes. You can then increase the time progressively. There are excellent guided meditation apps, which I will discuss later in this book.
- Be patient and compassionate with yourself and your teacher. Don't make any rash judgments!

Breathing meditation techniques

Those who have gained further experience in meditation sometimes choose a specific breathing technique during their meditation session. This is no obligation to do this, but it may prove beneficial as it allows for even better control over the way you breathe. I will now briefly talk you through a few of these techniques, although I would highly recommend that you are guided by a professional when you want to try them out.

This balanced breathing technique seems very natural, but in fact it follows a very specific rhythm. It is an ideal technique to reduce stress, stimulate concentration and hold one's nerve.

1. Inhale deeply through your nose while counting up to four.
2. Exhale deeply through your nose while counting up to four.
3. Repeat the exercise.

In contrast to the balanced breathing technique, which aims foremost at relaxation and soothing, this stimulating breathing technique allows you to be more energetic and alert.

1. Set your timer for three or five minutes.
2. As soon as you set it off, breathe through your nose and make sure that your inhalations and exhalations are as short as possible. Your inhalations and exhalations should be of the same duration.
3. Start breathing more slowly as soon as the timer stops, until you have returned to your normal rhythm of breathing.

Alternate nostril breathing may seem odd to start with, but it is a good technique to stimulate the brain and body. Beware that it is not ideal if you have a blocked nose!

1. Blow your nose and make sure you have entirely clear nostrils.
2. Raise your right arm. Close your fist, stick out your thumb and little finger. If you can't manage to keep your little finger straight, you can also raise your ring finger.
3. Place your thumb on your right nostril to hold it closed and inhale through your left nostril.
4. Pivot your hand slightly to liberate your right nostril and push in your left nostril. Then exhale slowly through your right nostril.
5. Inhale again deeply through your right nostril.
6. Pivot your hand slightly to liberate your left nostril and push in your right nostril. Then exhale through your left nostril.
7. Repeat the exercise and let yourself be carried away by the sensations you feel.

The 4-7-8 breathing technique is also called relaxation breathing. Breathing for a few minutes in this fashion is truly relaxing. It is actually often used by people who have trouble falling asleep.

1. Place the tip of your tongue behind your upper teeth.
2. Breathe out all the air in your lungs with a long and deep sigh.
3. Close your mouth and inhale deeply through your nose while counting to four.
4. Hold your breath while counting to seven.
5. Release all the air in your lungs again while counting to eight.
6. Repeat the whole cycle.

~

TESTIMONIAL: TIM PARKS

**'I was immediately extremely interested in the
meditative process, but at the time I didn't even know
it was meditation.'**

~

*Award-winning writer Tim Parks is the author of numerous novels, as well as
several non-fiction works. Although initially very resistant to the idea, he came
to meditation in a desperate attempt to deal with extreme physical pain. He
described his experience in his book,* Teach Us to Sit Still: A Sceptic's Search
for Health and Healing, *and he expands on that here, as well as telling us
how his practice has developed over the last 15 years.*

PRESSURE AND PAIN

To give some context, I was in my late 40s. I'd been living in Italy for about
20 years and working madly hard. I'd published more than 20 books and
was working as a professor at the university in Milan. I was translating and
living in two languages at once and I had three children, so I had a very
hectic and tense life. I started displaying a lot of symptoms of abdominal and
bladder pain, but a lot more pain than is normally associated with prostate
problems. I went to the urologist, as one does, and he did a lot of tests on
me and found that there was actually nothing wrong with my prostate. All
the same, he offered me an operation to open it up, as it were – the famous
TURP [transurethral resection of the prostate] operation – which I wisely
rejected. Then I went to see a very expensive urologist in London and he did
all the tests and, again, he told me that there was no serious problem that
he could identify and that he genuinely didn't know why I was in so much
pain. Although at the top of his profession, he acknowledged that there was
a situation he didn't recognise.

The pain was so considerable that I couldn't sit down for more than about
five minutes. I would stand up to write during the day and in the evening
half-lie on the sofa, and I was having to get up four or five, six times every

night to pee, but apart from that I was completely fit and even full of energy. I tried painkillers, which really didn't do very much. It's interesting, in the last 10 years a lot of literature has come out saying that 50 per cent of people with this condition enjoy a placebo effect with almost any medicine they take but I never had any placebo effect at all — never. If I took diazepam it did ease the symptoms at night, but at a big price, which I wasn't willing to pay. However, it's interesting that I had an operation on my foot during that period, which required a general anaesthetic, and for the 48 hours after that general anaesthetic I had no pain in my abdomen, even though the anaesthetic had apparently left my system, so it imposed on me a kind of deep relaxation that I needed.

After an enormous amount of research on the Internet, I luckily came across a guy called David Wise and a book called *A Headache in the Pelvis*. He had identified a syndrome, which is now officially recognised as Pelvic Pain Syndrome. Basically, the idea is you spend your whole life sitting tensely in a chair over a computer and your pelvic floor muscle tightens up. The nerves which cross that pelvic floor, from the prostate, from the bladder, from all kinds of other places, heading for your spinal cord, get constricted and you start getting what's called referred pain; that is, you start feeling pain in places that the pinched nerves go to, but the problem is actually in the pelvic floor.

So the problem, as it was presented by Dr Wise, was you've got to learn to relax very deeply and he had all kinds of solutions to this, including massage and anal massage in his clinic in California. But first of all, and most available, he suggested a series of relaxation exercises, which he called paradoxical relaxation. He suggested lying down, entering into reflex breathing and relaxing the muscles of the body deeply, and in particular the pelvic floor. I began to get some benefits almost immediately from this. It was remarkable. After all the doctors I'd been to, David Wise was the first guy who actually described all the symptoms that I had — and a few more that fortunately I didn't!

BREATHING EXERCISES

I was in pain and very, very anxious, which obviously makes things worse, for at least two years. Then I started doing these breathing exercises and I began to recognise that there was a sort of psychological profile, a way of behaving, which had led me to allow my body to reach this state. Above all, there was this sort of obsession with doing. I mean, I'm the kind of guy — or I used to be – who would never waste even two minutes of the day. I was immediately extremely interested in the meditative process, but at the time I didn't even know it was meditation. I'd been having shiatsu massages, and they were also extremely useful, and it was the guy doing the shiatsu massage who said to me, 'Look, what you're doing is basically meditation.' I was resistant to that, because I was brought up in a very religious household and I had rejected everything that had any hint of religion or mysticism.

So I resisted, but I was also very, very curious, and in the end my shiatsu practitioner encouraged me to go to a Vipassana meditation retreat. Vipassana is a very basic and very ancient form of meditation, and also a kind of a 'hard school of meditation'. I mean, it's not an easy entry. So about three years after all this began, I went to my first Vipassana meditation retreat and I've now been to one every year for the last 15 years, so usually 10-day retreats, or at least seven days.

At the beginning, I went to these relaxation methods to overcome a specific problem with the classic view that once that problem was overcome, as with taking any other medicine, I could stop bothering with this time-wasting business. What became clear immediately, with Vipassana meditation particularly, is that the practice will only work if you don't do it merely in order for it to work. If you take the view that this is a physical action in order to achieve a goal and leave it behind, you're not going to go very far. Gradually, I began to realise that what I needed to do was change my lifestyle, and then meditation became such an important, positive addition to my life that I continued anyway.

I think one of the problems with introducing meditation at a serious level in the West is it involves a profound invitation to change your life goals and to understand how much of your unease has to do with a certain kind of ambition, a certain kind of driven activity. So that was a really major turning point for me. Not that I left ambition behind, but I was able to get a lot more distance on it. I was able to step back from it, to see it more coolly, and have this other place that seemed more important and that in fact is more important.

REACTION FROM READERS

Teach Us to Sit Still became a bestseller and I had a really strong reaction from readers. Since I wrote it in 2010, I must have received a couple of thousand emails from people with the same condition. Obviously, anything that has to do with your bladder, that has to do with urination, is embarrassing and, when people have that kind of problem, they don't talk about it easily. As a result, the problem itself gets bigger, because they become more and more tense. Some people seriously contemplate suicide, because their pain just goes on and on, so I think there were a lot of people who just wanted to thank me for having put it out there.

When I wrote the first chapters of the book, my publisher said, 'Look, don't do this. Don't talk about stuff that's embarrassing and intimate, because you've got your career as a novelist and you don't want to be associated with it.' You can't imagine Ronaldo coming out and saying, 'I've got prostate problems,' or Donald Trump saying, 'I've got this issue with nocturnal urination.' It's not something that a winner does and a lot of the people who have pelvic pain syndrome are driven people who want to be winners, so a lot of *Teach Us to Sit Still* is about looking at our ambitions and looking at why we treat our bodies the way we treat them.

I always say to people, look, I tell this story in this book and I've moved on a long way from that. First of all, what people with this condition want to hear is that they're not going to die. Second, they want to hear that you can get better. Then I think it's useful for them to hear that in order to get better, they will probably have to examine their way of living quite deeply. I might suggest a book or two that they could look at and maybe a website or two that they might go to, but I think that's enough input from me. When I began this I wasn't ready to start meditating immediately and when people contact me I think it's important not to encourage them to do things that they might not be ready to do. So I say, look, there's this experience I've had. Maybe someday you'll want to try it.

MEDITATION PRACTICE

My partner and I meditate for 45 minutes, not absolutely every morning, we try not to make it a prison, but we probably do it five days a week, and then we go to retreats where one meditates for maybe eight hours a day. What I find extraordinary about the meditation process is that even though I've been doing it for 15 years now, I still consider myself a beginner. It's a constantly changing thing and you learn, maybe like peeling an onion, that what you thought was relaxed before, was really not. And then again, what you think is relaxed now, is really not. There's always a deeper and deeper place to go, and that deeper place always comes together with a newly learned attitude.

Let's say there are these positions of the mind, or behaviours, which you learn in meditation, but which, because they're not visible, are very difficult to describe. All that people teaching you meditation can do is suggest a number of techniques and approaches and attitudes, but it's only when you experience different depths of absorption that you say, 'Aha, so that's what they meant.' Establishing how long you plan to meditate is important in this regard. If you don't put a timer on, for example, you're going to be constantly faced with the decision of when to stop, and once you're faced with that decision, you can't meditate, so I use a timer. I have a nice little gong timer on my computer, which is softer than an alarm, and you don't have to switch it off, so that if you don't want to stop when the gong goes off, you don't have to.

One of the interesting things about meditation and Buddhism is the teaching of non-attachment. It's a difficult teaching for people who grew up with the background I did, because it doesn't mean a cynical detachment, but a learning to accept that things end and that when they end you might suffer, but that doesn't mean you can't enjoy them now. Sometimes when I was in a meditation retreat, the gong would go to end the hour and I would be upset, because I was really deeply in it and I wanted to go on, and then I realised that this too is another form of attachment – best let it go – the moment was beautiful, but it was over.

I can't sit in a lotus position, although I can sit in a Burmese position, with the two legs next to each other. I used to get a lot of pain sitting in that position and one of the interesting things about meditation is how it can induce the kind of pain you want to learn to deal with. Until you get used to it, for a lot of people sitting in a cross-legged position will induce severe pain. For most people – though this is something you need to check – that pain is inconsequential, it goes the minute you move, but

I learned very early on that if I'm focused on the breathing, the observing and the deep relaxation, that pain will defuse. As a result the transitory pains of the sitting position become an inducement to the practice. Honestly, this is something that people can't understand unless they've done it – I couldn't and it took me a few years – but when you arrive in a deep state of absorption, sitting in with a straight back in the cross-legged position, it is a beautiful experience.

For me, meditation has been nothing other than learning the process of being there and observing. In Vipassana they have this expression 'entering the flow', where you basically get a sense that the self is simply being absorbed into a stream of observation. You retain the ability to snap out of it if you want to, but I suppose one of the curious things is the extent to which, on the one hand, there's a relinquishing of control, and on the other hand, it's a practice of control. When you go to a retreat, you go into much deeper levels of absorption, into the sound of the world around you or what's going on in your body. There are an enormous number of things going on in your body that you have very little awareness of normally and that begin to emerge with meditation. I have a friend who meditates a lot and concentrating very slowly on the parts of his body he became aware that there were things happening that he wasn't used to, so he went to the doctor and found he had a tumour, due to his awareness of what was going on when he was meditating.

FASCINATED BY BUDDHISM

Buddhism interests me a lot, but I haven't become a Buddhist and even the question seems to be the wrong sort of question. As far as I know, Buddhism doesn't require you to make declarations of belief. Buddhism is an invitation to observe life in a certain way and follow certain practices, but you don't have to sign up to all of them. The retreats that I go to are run by Buddhist organisations, but what I love about Buddhism, unlike the evangelical religion I grew up in, is that there is no attempt to proselytise. Nobody ever says, 'Isn't it time you became a Buddhist?'

As far as I know, the belief in reincarnation is not a necessary part of Buddhism, nor do Buddhists speak specifically about the need to believe in stuff like that. I certainly don't believe in it. Christianity offers eternal life, in return for, as it were, a belief in the identity of Christ and the nature of his sacrifice, but there's really none of that in Buddhism. Similarly, karma is a description of what the self is over a period of time and if you believe in reincarnation you might accept that your karma finds its way into some other being. This is mystical speculation, but karma is an interesting way to describe what we mean by the self, because it's clear that the self is not a static thing; that there is an accumulation of behaviours and memories, and also a loss of behaviours and memories. It's an accumulation of what you've been and what you've done, and that's probably a better description than just saying, 'I'm Tim Parks... I was Tim Parks when I was five... I was Tim Parks when I was 40.' I'm clearly very different from what I was at 40 and certainly from what I was when I was five or 10.

CREATIVITY AND CHANGE

How has meditation influenced me as an artist, a writer, a creative person? It's a difficult question. Obviously, it influences you in every way, but nothing you could immediately point to in this or that sentence. I suppose most of all it reminded me not to be too attached to success and to take more pleasure in the actual process of making art, of writing well — to just enjoy it. You reach a point where it's not that you don't care, but you know that this or that bad news could spoil your lunch but it's not going to spoil your dinner! The important thing is that I'm here now, reasonably physically well and I'm happy — and that's actually quite a lot.

The creative process, like any other living process, changes all the time, but I think this experience has changed the kind of stories that I find myself telling. I wrote a series of books, one book called *Europa*, which was shortlisted for the Booker Prize, and a book called *Destiny*, which was very successful in Germany. These are books that end in a profound psychological dead end with no way out, and I just don't feel like that about life anymore, so I don't write those books anymore. I write books that might be full of tension and difficulty, but they're not going to finish in a dead end, so things do change. Funnily enough, I had some emails from readers who were disappointed that I'm not as pessimistic as I used to be!

~

Chapter 8

Mindfulness here and now

~

'Mindfulness is not difficult, we just
need to remember to do it.'

– SHARON SALZBERG, Co-founder of the Insight Meditation Society

Why does time fly once we are adults? I am sure this question must have occurred to you too. As a child, the hours seemed to pass much more slowly. Back then, time seemed infinite, a bit like the prairies that stretched as far the eye could see in the cowboy stories that our parents would tell us. Now, some decades later, the hours are as fleeting as the fine sand that slips through our fingers. How is that possible? In fact, the answer is quite simple. It is all a matter of state of mind and way of thinking. As a young child you used to live only in the present. What happened the night before didn't really matter and the future didn't mean anything tangible to you. As long as you were fed when you were hungry and changed when needed, everything was fine. This is what I admire so much when I watch my son, three-year-old Louis. He never gets lost in memories, nor does he build any long-term plans for the future. All that matters to him is what stimulates his curiosity and makes him marvel there and then. When he grows into an adult, he will understand that he has already lived many years of his life and that his time is limited. He will cherish his memories, but most of all he will want to make projects for the future. Awareness of past and future comes hand and in hand with a greater sense of responsibility, and by the same token of time constraints. Just like his father, he will be aware of these time constraints, which explains why as adults we have the impression that time flies by like a high-speed train. And for that reason, we organise our lives and holidays on a very precise and tight schedule.

When we travel, we keep calculating how much time we need to reach the next appointment or tourist attraction instead of enjoying the beauty that surrounds us in the very place we are. After the holidays are over, we tend to reminisce about the lovely moments we have experienced. In a nutshell, we tend to forget to be happy here and now. And I am speaking from experience. During a recent trip to Canada I went climbing with my son Matias, then 13 years old. The rock was next to a magnificent waterfall. Hanging by my rope, I wanted at all costs to take several pictures of him. I was adamant about providing Matias with a tangible memory of the moment. It didn't take long before he got really annoyed with having me behind him like the paparazzi. He turned around towards me and I will never forget what he said to me: 'Dad, when are you going to put away that camera of yours and admire the landscape around you? Look how beautiful it is! Enjoy it!' Of course, he was spot on. My teenager called me back to the obvious. I was hanging by a rope, I was surrounded by the splendours of nature, and the only thing that mattered to me was to capture in pictures for later the spectacle that I was missing out on in the present moment. Mindfulness is just about that: living the present moment, here and now; becoming aware of oneself, of what surrounds us, of the lived moment and the unique quality of happiness each brings.

I think therefore I am, as the saying goes, but our modern lifestyles are full of responsibilities and stresses, and in our daily lives we are constantly made to look both forwards and backwards, with looming deadlines to abide by, endless meetings to sit through, and reductions for early bookings that we must not miss out on etc... In the long run our minds become so bogged down by detail that we become oblivious to the fact that our 'monkey mind' is constantly wandering. Day and night our thoughts run through our mind without us being able to control them. In

Our minds become so bogged down by detail that we become oblivious to the fact that our 'monkey mind' is constantly wandering.

effect, our brain behaves like a rather dull football commentator when the actual match is breath-taking. And instead of focusing on the match, we are distracted by our internal voice. But there is good news! Mindfulness can silence the voice of that undesirable commentator!

Mindfulness is the ultimate tool to train your mind to be fully aware of the present moment and to enjoy the here and now. What I like about mindfulness is that you can flexibly adapt its principles. You can do it formally, and I will come back to this form of mindfulness and guide you through it later in this chapter. But you can also apply it in your everyday life. You can, for example, make a habit of enjoying a nice cup of coffee or tea in full awareness, rather than gulping it down while preparing the documents that you need to take to work. Or you can take the time to enjoy the scents and noises around you, and admire the landscape, on a Sunday afternoon walk, rather than mentally preparing all you need to do during the week. Or decide knowingly what you will be buying at the supermarket there and then, rather than randomly piling items into your trolley with your mind elsewhere...

I am sure you're thinking that this is easier said than done and I am not going to contradict you. I was very much a restless control freak myself and I'm often reminded of this by my wife and kids. As I confessed, when on holiday, I may at times be too busy keeping a close eye on our timing and snapping away with my camera to capture the beauty of the moment, of the people or the landscape. Professionally as well, I was inclined to take the shortcut and get ahead of myself. And in the evening I would gulp down the meal my wife had lovingly cooked – just as my dog does! – while being unable to recall or tell you what I just had. That is a pity, because my wife is a brilliant cook. And it is precisely because it isn't easy to live consciously and enjoy the present moment on an everyday basis that I'd like to encourage you to develop this kind of awareness by using mindfulness techniques, whether formal or informal. If I can do it, anyone can do it. Mindfulness meditation allows us to create states of conscious awareness, which in turn allow us to change our state of mind in our everyday life more easily, to hush that sometimes annoying commentator and to create the impression that time passing can be enjoyed more slowly, more intensely and with enhanced appreciation.

Mindfulness meditation is a technique that can be learnt by all of us. It helps us achieve better self-awareness and knowledge of how the mind works, which in turn allows us to progressively change our state of mind. Mindfulness, however, is not only about having enhanced awareness of oneself and one's environment. It also entails taking stock without judging. To train for mindfulness also means to train to stop assessing, comparing, analysing, criticising and judging. And because you will no longer categorise your experiences as being good or bad, appropriate or inappropriate, to a certain extent mindfulness will help you to open your mind.

In other words, you will become much more receptive and attentive to who you are and where you are, simply because you will no longer waste energy on useless analyses and you will be much more mindful of small details that otherwise would have been lost upon you. It is one thing to know what mindfulness is about, what it entails and how it can be beneficial, but, most importantly, you need to practise it. Let's start with a short and very simple exercise that might allow you to grasp what mindfulness is really about.

Look for a photo of yourself with your friends or loved ones, whether it's on your smartphone or in an album. Set your timer for two or three minutes. The point of the exercise is to look attentively at the picture and observe all the elements represented without judging them. Here are a few tips. Look carefully at all the people who are on the picture. How are they dressed? What are their facial expressions? What do you see in the background? Be careful, the aim is not to judge what you see. Now close this book and try it out. You can come back to the book and find out whether you did the exercise correctly once you are done.

Two minutes have passed — and you may have felt that they lasted forever. Perfect! This means you have just succeeded in doing your first mindfulness exercise. But let's have a more detailed debrief. Did you really manage to remain focused on what you could see in the picture during the two minutes? If so, congratulations, you have been attentive. Did you think only about the exercise and the visual image or did your thoughts wander? If so, you may not have been that focused after all. You weren't focused if you passed judgment on Aunt Rita's dress or the weather you had that day, if the picture called up nice memories or if you told yourself that you were much slimmer then than now. But if you realised at some point that your thoughts were straying and you managed to refocus your attention on the picture, that means you succeeded in being attentive again.

If you beat yourself up over the fact that your thoughts strayed and if you started mulling over the fact that you did the exercise incorrectly, then you forgot to be attentive again. But if you realised that you were in the process of judging yourself for having these thoughts, then you were attentive again. In a nutshell, it doesn't matter whether your thoughts wandered off or you made any form of judgment, the important thing is that you were able to refocus your attention on your target. The more you do the exercise, the easier you will find it not to heed the thoughts that go through your mind, not to analyse them and not to judge, and the more you will also be able to remain focused on your target.

As soon as you understand what it's all about, you will be able to apply mindfulness meditation in various different ways: as short or long sessions, while sitting down or walking around, formally or informally, alone or as a group... I shall help you with this by suggesting a few easy exercises you can do!

Let's get started!

At the beginning of the book, I asked you to take the time to relish a piece of chocolate or a cup of tea. This is a classic exercise for beginners in mindfulness meditation. In principle, you can do the longer version of this exercise with any type of food, but certainly choosing one with a distinctive smell, texture and taste will make the exercise much easier. Raisins will therefore do the job perfectly.

The purpose is to engage all your senses in order to eat your raison mindfully. You will do so by focusing your attention on the following questions:

1. What does this raisin look like?
2. What do you feel when you touch it? What happens when you squeeze it, roll it or pull it?
3. What scent does it release?
4. What sensation do you have when you put it on your lips, your tongue and when you have it in your mouth?
5. What does it taste like?

To clarify, the aim is to formulate answers that do not express a judgment. For instance, in answer to the question, 'What scent does it release?', you might say 'a sweet smell' rather than 'a pleasant smell'.

The next exercise is a body scan, which consists of focusing on the different sensations in your body. It is not my favourite exercise, but it is one of the best known and most popular mindfulness techniques. My wife and my eldest daughter Clara love this exercise as it helps them relax before going to sleep. This exercise enhances not only awareness, but also the connection between mind and body. It is often recommended to those who suffer from physical disorders and chronic pain. The practice of mindfulness meditation does not cause pain to disappear as such, but it allows you to relate differently to it. In other words, the exercise encourages you to accept the sensations that you feel in the different parts of the body. These sensations then become more bearable as you choose to consciously reduce the suffering caused by chronic pain.

1. Lie down on your back with the palms of your hands turned upwards and your feet slightly apart. Close your eyes. If you're afraid you'll fall asleep you may prefer to do the body scan sitting up. In which case, sit on a chair with your back straight and your feet flat on the floor.

2. Whether you're lying or sitting, try to remain as still as you can. Only change position if you feel uncomfortable, sore or have any other issues, and move your body very slowly, in a conscious way. Think about the movements you are doing and the position you want to take up in order to be more comfortable.

3. Start to breathe mindfully. You do not need to apply any technique in particular, just focus on your breathing. This will help you relax and calm down before you start the exercise.

4. As soon as you feel calm, stop focusing on your breathing and turn to your body. What sensations can you identify? Do you feel the clothes you are wearing? Where is your body in touch with the floor? Do you feel hot or cold? Does your body feel relaxed or are your muscles tense?

5. Once you feel comfortable in your body, you have two options. You can either focus your attention progressively on the different parts of your body, starting with your toes and going up to the top of your skull. In that case, take stock of all the sensations in each of these parts and ask yourself whether you could change the way you experience that sensation. If you need more time, or if you want to do a body scan that is more focused, you may want to choose a body part that is more tense, tingles, or feels heavier or sorer. Do one side of your body after the other. Try to relax these parts with full awareness. It is in the here and now that you need to let go or accept the sensation of discomfort, so that you don't suffer it any longer.

6. After two to 10 minutes, once you have investigated all the regions of your body and feel that your body is more relaxed, open your eyes and linger in that comfortable position for a little while. Do you feel you are much more aware of your body and the connection between your body and mind?

Me and them

As well as the survival instinct we all have that I mentioned earlier, we also all have to face a certain duality. We tend to distinguish ourselves from the world that surrounds us: there is 'me' and 'them'. We also tend to feel angry at other people and then we tend to forget that in fact this 'me and them' forms a single whole. What's more, our brain often tells us to get personally involved, when in fact there is nothing personal in the situation at hand. Remember, for instance, when you were young, how your best friend got told off for something he hadn't done and how enraged you were by that. This duality within human beings also stirs up a lot of negative activity in the brain. We also live in a constantly changing world and we evolve constantly. This can be rather frustrating since as human beings we have been trained to seek stability and balance. We often want to have control over our lives, to plan, orchestrate and give them a clearly delineated shape. This might all be in vain! It is impossible to control every single thing. We can't prevent natural disasters, the provocations inflicted on us by our teenage kids, our colleagues or neighbours, the lines and wrinkles that grow deeper on our brow, or the fact that our houseplant will give up the ghost sooner or later.

The trick, then, is to accept and understand the fact that as human beings we all act in a certain way and that we cannot control everyone around us. You will not necessarily be in a position to quickly change jobs when your boss is harassing you, to move if you can't take the North Sea climate any longer or to have any control over your teenage kid when he is going through his rebellion phase. However, what you do have control over is the way you deal with situations. A great deal of your 'suffering' is therefore in your hands.

Allow me to illustrate this with a simple example: a traffic jam. You didn't anticipate it, so it's perfectly understandable that you become irritated, but the question is where will this irritation get you? The truth is nowhere. On the contrary, you won't be able to change anything about the situation. No one intentionally wants to irritate you and, in fact, you alone are responsible for your exasperation. Instead, why not accept the situation for what it is and try to take advantage of it in the best way you can? Play your favourite piece of music, turn up the volume, and sing along with the artist that you like so much. With a little luck, you will recall good memories from the concert you attended, the song you enjoyed so much at your wedding party or the great evening you had the previous weekend. Or call your loved ones, listen to an audio book or – and why not? – do some meditation...

The same goes for your interactions with others. Allow me again to give you a simple illustration. After work you decide to quickly swing by the supermarket. Of course, there are long queues at the tills. You quickly gauge which of them is going fastest and join it. In the end, things don't happen as you want them to and the people in the queue next to you, who arrived after you, are getting to the till much quicker and finish their shopping before you. This could be really irritating. You could even get angry with the other customers or the cashier, who isn't working fast enough. Your brain fills with negative thoughts and emotions. But what about not stressing over it anymore? Just be happy for the people in the other queue and empathise with those, like you, who chose the wrong one. After all, none of you chose to wait, but you are all stuck with it. Take some deep calming breaths and let go of your negative thoughts and emotions. In fact, it is possible to live mindfully: to eat, drink, communicate and even do the housework mindfully.

It is all about simply being more aware when you interact with others. The next time you talk to someone, do really take the time to talk and focus on the person, rather than going into autopilot mode. When you wake up, don't jump out of bed, but enjoy the present moment.

Mindfulness in eight weeks or 10 days

When I prescribe meditation or mindfulness sessions for my patients, I first refer them to a qualified psychologist or a traditional mindfulness-based stress reduction (MBSR) group, which is typically planned around nine sessions, varying from a few hours to a full day, and carried out over eight weeks. As I was prescribing these sessions, it seemed only fair that I should follow the programme myself, and so I enrolled together with my wife and part of the team at my clinic. At the start of the programme all participants usually introduce themselves, say who they are and where they come from. This may sound a bit like an Alcoholics Anonymous meeting and some participants sometimes have quite a poignant life story to tell. Others may be patients who suffer from a very specific condition and some may simply be curious or be healthcare professionals. Just like the other participants, I tried out all sorts of exercises, ranging from yoga, breathing exercises, exercises focusing on sensory experiences, exercises like focusing on a raisin or a lit candle. I also had tasks to fulfil, such as the pebble for my pocket exercise, which consists of putting a pebble in your pocket without looking at it. The aim is to touch the pebble from time to time. I discovered to my great surprise that the virtual reality machine in my mind was all too happy to literally invent the characteristics of the pebble. I started to imagine all sorts of colours and shapes without ever having seen it.

Sometimes during the training I would suddenly be overwhelmed by an unpleasant feeling of doubt. 'Here I am, a responsible adult able to take care of myself, playing with a raisin or a pebble in my pocket.' But once I had overcome that doubt and decided to go along with the game, the training suddenly became very interesting and fulfilling. I learnt that mindfulness is not about focusing on a symptom or anything else specifically, but that it's about observation, and letting go and accepting without judging. At times, I felt pervaded by scepticism, yet the aim is not to try to think of nothing at any cost, but, on the contrary, to note one's thoughts and feelings, let go of them. This can be very rewarding in our stressful environment, in which overstimulation puts our capacity to think and plan at risk.

This same capacity to worry can also stop us from sleeping, as falling asleep requires us to let go. The harder you try, the less it works. This is how I learnt that mindfulness is not only an exercise in 'dropping it', but also in acceptance. If thoughts enter your mind while you are meditating, don't be disappointed. Just take stock and don't judge. This may seem simple, but in fact it isn't.

Apart from my MBSR training, I also did a number of meditation retreats. If you believe that a retreat is like a 'Club Med' type of holiday village, you will be disappointed, for as Matthieu would say, 'Meditation is not entertainment.' During my first retreat, at the Mind & Life Europe summer school in 2014, I also discovered forms of meditation that I found less attractive, like walking meditation. I must confess that walking over a distance of a few metres at an extremely slow pace made me feel totally ridiculous. We also spent long moments in silence and, as my partner was there with me, it felt strange not to be able to talk to her. We also had to adapt to the monks' style: they would be talking to you and then, when they banged their gong, they would suddenly enter into silence for some time. You would then be left to your own devices.

I have to admit that I found that very difficult, but the periods of silence during these retreats are not really a matter of discipline. When your brain is immersed in silence, after a while you naturally become more mindful of yourself if you are meditating or more mindful of the environment if you are out for a walk. We know that the senses activate different brain networks. When one sense is not engaged, the other senses will be quick to take over the mind space that has freed up. That's why a person who has become blind will, over time, develop an enhanced sense of taste, hearing or touch. My wife and I were able to experience this first hand in an extraordinary way when we went to the blind people's restaurant in Montreal. When we arrived, the venue was dimmed to almost darkness and a blind person came to guide us towards our table. We took our seats fumbling about. We did not really know what we would be eating. There were only two options on offer, the adventure set menu or the wise set menu. We went for the adventure one. We were served several dishes and I hadn't the foggiest idea what I was sticking in my mouth. I could hardly tell whether it was chicken or pork, tofu or meat? Even when I was sipping my wine, I could not identify for sure whether it was red or white. My wife's ability for blind tasting was clearly much better than mine. At the end of the meal we were told what we had eaten. The supposed tofu was in fact brains and it has to be said that eating brains is far more daring than having tofu.

Despite the challenge it represented, that first meditation retreat did make me want to do more. In the autumn of 2018, I put my mobile phone into flight mode and took off to a retreat in the beautiful castle and Tibetan temple Yeunten Ling, which means Garden of Qualities, located in Huy,

Belgium! I warned everyone at the hospital and at the lab that I would be on leave and unreachable for four days. That alone felt like a great relief! The retreat there was an incredible experience. My host Lama Zeupa seemed, like all the other Buddhist monks that I met, the very incarnation of quietude and wisdom. My wife sometimes jokes saying that it is easy enough for a lama to let go since he does not need to do the shopping, go to work or take care of the children... Not only does Lama Zeupa enjoy a mind in excellent condition, he has also developed a perfect body thanks to years of intense training in CrossFit. Every day, we kicked off with a yoga session coached by Chookela, Zeupa's sister, and a solid vegan breakfast, followed by a vigorous walk in the woods. After that the programme featured several meditation sessions, as well as various theoretical teachings. The lessons that Lama Zeupa taught and which drew on Buddhist philosophy have been a true source of inspiration.

There were always three meditation sessions. Between each, we would have a break to stretch and shake our legs. In the beginning, we would exchange a few words and ask a few questions in a low voice, but over time these breaks became more and more silent. You always had to wait for the gong to know when the next session was starting and you didn't know its duration in advance, but we spent long hours meditating. It was a very intense experience, during which I sometimes asked myself what I was doing there.

I still have a perfectly clear recollection of the first session. We started off with a short 10-minute meditation session as a warm-up. That may seem ridiculously short, but when you are sitting in an awkward lotus position, your nose is itching and your knees hurt, it feels like an eternity. Between two sessions, I casually mentioned to the Lama that my knees were horrendously painful. 'Fantastic,' he replied. 'Use your pain, observe it... You are not your pain.' I took my cue from his good advice and focused on the nature of the painful sensation, and I indeed realised that it wavered between intense pain and a total absence of it.

Lama Zeupa was a wonderful, accommodating and indulgent guide. We became friends and I invited him (as I had Matthieu) to be a guinea pig in our lab. I have returned to his Tibetan Buddhist institute many times since.

I later learned Zeupa means 'patient' – just the quality I needed from my meditation teacher.

One single task

Over the last few years, mindfulness has become very fashionable. At times I have felt that this rich contemplative tradition has been shredded for commercial benefits and that only a superficial version of it has survived. Admittedly, this may seem exaggerated, but as with any other trend to do with health, it is important to bring in nuance and caution.

Despite being a fashionable phenomenon, meditation and mindfulness are also a way of being or, rather, an attempt at being. To practise it, you do not need to spend hours on end sitting on a small rug. It is an exercise that you can do while cooking or doing the dishes. There are a great variety of exercises on offer and I have given you a taste of some of them in this book. For instance, you may want to take in the splendours of a landscape in full awareness or investigate an emotion as you experience it in the moment. The main idea remains the same: turn off autopilot mode and focus on the present moment, the here and now. We always want to do a thousand things at once instead of investing in one thing at a time, or even doing nothing.

In that respect, a study carried out by Stanford University[1] has shown that multitasking is a myth. Our brain is not really able to do several things that all require real concentration at once. Our mind simply hops very quickly from one task to another and thus uses more cognitive energy. New technologies are ubiquitous in our daily lives and they are very useful, but various studies carried out on keen users of a multiplicity of media all reveal that subjects score poorer results on tasks involving long-term, focused attention. And what is most ironic is that they are slower at moving on from one task to the next! In a nutshell, as Matthieu would say, 'The tendency to multi-task just creates a disorderly mind and brain!'

You don't believe me? Or my Stanford colleagues? Then please do the following simple experiment. Take a sheet of paper and draw two horizontal lines. On the first, write the following sentence: I believe it is possible to do several tasks at the same time. On the second line, write the first fifteen letters of the alphabet: a b c d e f g h i j k l m n o.

How long did it take you? Often it takes about 20 seconds. Now, let's try and do several things at the same time. Take a sheet of paper and draw two horizontal lines. Write the first letter of the sentence above on the first line and the first letter of the alphabet on the second line. Then write the second letter of the sentence on the first line and the second letter of the alphabet on the second line. Do it until you have completed the sentence.

'I b...'

'a b...'

The chances are that you will give up quickly. And I don't blame you. Not only is it time-consuming, the second part of the exercise is also clearly more difficult and unbelievably dull.

TESTIMONIAL: EDEL MAEX

'It is possible to strike the right balance between fleeing reality, on the one hand, and letting oneself be overtaken by grief and sadness on the other!'

~

My colleague and friend Edel Maex is a psychiatrist, whereas I am a neurologist. In a nutshell, we both work with mental and brain illnesses and, in my view at least, psychiatry is just a subset of neurology that we have not yet been able to understand. As a pioneer in mindfulness training, Edel is the author of several bestsellers on the topic.[2] He runs a stress clinic, where for many years he has been fully committed to treating his patients by using mindfulness as a therapy. As you will see when you read our discussion, the man is a shining example of integrity and wisdom!

PERSONAL JOURNEY

Meditation is a rather baggy notion. When I hear someone talk about it, I always ask for clarification about what he or she means. Meditation can indeed be interpreted in various ways. It is a bit like a toolbox that you can fill as you wish. I started meditating when I was going through a rather difficult patch. I had just finished my studies and I needed to move on with my life. I was trying to escape the grief caused by a breakup and was throwing myself into new relationships. The challenges attached to the profession of psychiatrist were also a main contributing factor. How to deal with the pain of others? All medics suffer from post-traumatic stress disorder, because they are confronted with the pain of others. How to keep your head above the water when you are going through a difficult spell on an emotional level? My strategy was to flee everything that really worried me. I needed not to think about my sadness. I was partying like mad and literally it was mad. My attitude only made things worse, until a friend of mine suggested I confront my own sadness. I spontaneously told him I could not, but as I was up against the wall, I tried nevertheless and luckily my friend was always there to offer his support.

To my great surprise, I did not fall apart when I faced up to my sadness. On the contrary, facing my emotions was a very meaningful experience. I should specify, though, that all this happened without me doing any mindfulness. A while later, I happened to meet a Dutch Zen master who repeated the same message: don't ignore your emotions, try to face up to them. I then had a revelation! It is possible to strike the right balance between fleeing reality, on the one hand, and letting oneself be overtaken by grief and sadness on the other! And for me that right balance was to be found in meditation. I took up meditation with a Zen group that gathered once a week. At some point the group dispersed, but I nevertheless continued to meditate. During the first year I did it, I didn't read up on the topic, which was surprising since I normally delve into a discipline at an intellectual level first, before putting it into practice. For meditation I did the opposite and it was really stimulating to be able to recognise in my reading what I had already experienced by myself!

WITH REGARD TO BUDDHISM

I started meditating in the context of Zen Buddhism, even though I do not consider myself either a Buddhist or an atheist. Even the title of professor is problematic to me, because it has a connotation I don't feel comfortable with. That being said, I have read extensively on the topic and my personal library is full of books on Buddhism, but the fact remains that I don't feel comfortable being labelled a Buddhist. Conflating religion and personal identity is a characteristic of monotheism and the three Abrahamic religions that settled around the Mediterranean. This conflation rests on the biblical notion that there is an alliance between God and his people. In the Asian countries, very few will identify as Buddhists. Neither in India or China are people familiar with this conflation of religion and personal identity. I am very interested in Buddhism and I often use it as a reference in my work, but I don't specifically follow one of its traditions over another. Buddha inspires me as a clear-sighted and pragmatic mind. In that respect, for instance, I don't believe in reincarnation. I have had several discussions on this. My understanding of karma is also different. Literally, karma means 'attitude' in the behavioural sense. Buddha says that we are all responsible for our own behaviour and therefore for the consequences it has. In that respect, I do believe that the concept of karma is useful, but that our good actions should have an influence on our afterlife does not make sense to me at all.

What I like very much in the Zen tradition is its core principle — the belief that we all already have in us what we are looking for. If a mindfulness programme yields results over just eight weeks, this is precisely because people work with what is already in them! Otherwise these programmes would not be as quick and effective. People don't really learn mindfulness they learn how to recognise it. They don't learn something new they learn to recognise something that already exists in each of them.

RETREATS

When I started practising meditation, I did not much like going on retreats. I found it all a bit over the top. But as time went by, I began to develop an urge for them. When my children were young, my retreats would be limited to a few days, as I didn't want to leave them alone for too long. Now I organise several retreats a year for myself. It is important to be able to dedicate time to them. I generally choose retreats of at least three days as I personally find two days too short. Formal practice consists of practising sitting and walking meditation in complete silence. As it happens, I have had the opportunity to take part in a disciplined and rigorous retreat that lasted over seven days, but I have now realised that such rigour did not yield much. To a certain extent it was counter-productive and meditation threatened to become what it is not. Effort is always energising. Running a marathon or climbing the Everest generate a release of adrenaline, and after a demanding retreat you will feel the same, but you will be straying from the core principle of what a retreat is about.

EAST AND WEST

I love travelling and I often visited Asian countries. However, most of the knowledge I have gathered on meditation comes from Europe. In Asia, you will often find that Buddhist rituals are replete with incense sticks and cards, but that doesn't mean that people meditate a lot. In fact, I have found relatively little of what constitutes the essence of meditation for me in those countries.

Last summer, I had a very interesting conversation on this topic with a woman I met in Kathmandu. She had married a European and had had an international career. During her youth, she had been nourished by Buddhist rituals, temples and festivals, but she had never really distinguished between

Hinduism and Buddhism. It was only recently that she had discovered the theory that underpinned the rituals. Oddly, in the West, we always start by studying the theory before discovering the rest. I have also discovered subsequently that Zen practices are not homogenous and that meditation is a crucial element in certain Buddhist traditions, but less so in others. It is said that mindfulness is a Christian practice. In a sense that is not really wrong, but it is also a Buddhist practice. Fundamentally, meditation is not linked to a religion.

MINDFULNESS AS THERAPY

After 10 years or so of practice, I started to think about the ways in which mindfulness and meditation could feed into my work as a psychiatrist. Both had helped me and I could now in turn help others by teaching them. I often saw patients painfully conflicted, lost in their grief and perceiving themselves as the enemy. One of the greatest problems of our culture today is that people suffer from a total lack of self-esteem and they internalise the violence they are confronted with. That is why I wanted to teach meditation, even though I had no clue how to go about it. That's when I discovered that Jon Kabat-Zinn, the founder of the Stress Reduction Clinic at the University of Massachusetts, had developed a similar stress reduction programme based on mindfulness (MBSR). At that time there was no formal training, so I contacted him directly and he suggested that I use my last 10 years of personal experience in meditation.

In 2005, in the whirl of life, I wrote *Mindfulness*, my first book on the topic, based on the notes of my sessions. To start with I had reservations about publishing them as I had not taken them for that purpose, but in the end the book sold over 100,000 copies. Today only cookery books sell in those numbers!

I am currently director of a stress clinic in Antwerp where everything we undertake is linked to mindfulness. I run an eight-week programme inspired by MBSR and to date I have organised 280 of these. The programme took shape over time, but I still draw on what I learnt from the first sessions I did with my Zen group. The eight-week programme has proved successful, but eight weeks is not a golden rule as strict norms are one of the pitfalls mindfulness seeks to avoid. In truth, what is paramount is the quality of attention and many structures can be used to attain that quality. I often use learning to swim as a metaphor. Most of us know how to swim, even though we have never been taught. A human being floats by default, since you have to empty your lungs in order to go underwater, so in order to learn how to swim you first need to understand that the human body floats. That is what I mean when I say the capacity already lies in us (Buddhists would say that it is Buddha that we already have in us). The first step entails trusting that we will float, so we don't panic once we enter the water. The second step entails learning how to travel forward. That's all there is to know. Of course, you can train for the Olympics if you want to, but that's not really necessary if you just want to learn how to swim... Likewise, there are several ways of learning how to enhance your attention. I have never used any apps, but I have heard lots of good things about Headspace.

MEDICATION, MINDFULNESS AND PSYCHOTHERAPY

Psychiatrists have several tools at their disposal to aid their patients: medication, mindfulness and psychotherapy. At the risk of being simplistic, medication essentially stops the development of the illness and can therefore be useful at times, but today I very rarely prescribe medication. It is not that I am against it on principle, but I don't prescribe them. If anti-depressants are necessary, I ask patients to talk to their GP. Psychotherapy is there to give meaning to what has happened to patients and explore the roots of their suffering. When it comes to mindfulness or meditation, however, it is neither about the history or the suppression of symptoms: it is about managing what happens. Mindfulness, as far as I am concerned, has become a 'super-specialism', but the three treatments are not mutually exclusive and a number of patients have benefited from combining all three.

The patients I work with present with very diverse types of pathologies. Some suffer from depression, burnout, anxiety or chronic fatigue. I don't treat patients who suffer from extreme psychiatric disorders as these would indeed require a much more specialised approach, particularly if you are dealing with psychoses, and Professor Paul Chadwick, who is based in the UK, is a specialist in these matters. Psychotic and schizophrenic patients don't come to me, but in principle it is possible to incorporate forms of mindfulness into their treatment as long as it is done in the appropriate context. Others who suffer from non-clinical stress disorders come to see us often out of sheer curiosity. Working on quality of attention, whatever the treatment, is always useful, but for some the traditional eight-week programme is too long and doing the exercises every day may sometimes simply prove too difficult.

MEDICINE, RESEARCH AND MINDFULNESS

I don't do research on mindfulness, but I believe we need to develop this and we need more researchers who are passionate about it. At the University of Antwerp, medical students are lucky enough to have courses in mindfulness from their first year through to their sixth. For instance, they become familiar with the three minutes' breathing space exercise, which they find very useful. Recently, we invited Ron Epstein to give a lecture at the university. This GP, who is a firm believer in Zen meditation, has written *Attending*,[3] a book I highly recommend to all doctors and medical students. The book has a pragmatic approach and broaches numerous everyday situations. For instance, a patient steps through your door and you don't know what to tell him...

MINDFULNESS AND TRANSCENDENTAL MEDITATION

Transcendental meditation differs totally from mindfulness as I practise it. In this type of meditation you need to extract yourself from the reality around you with the help of mantras (which also exist in Buddhism). This might seem strange to some, but it is a pure relaxation technique. Conversely, the key principle of mindfulness and of Zen practice is not to extract oneself from reality, but to focus all one's attention on it. Mindfulness does things differently. They are just two different strands. It is a bit like volleyball and football: they are not mutually exclusive, but you can't practise them at the same time. The same is true for yoga. Some practise it to connect with their own body, others to take care of it, while others use it for relaxation. They are all techniques that have their own purpose and own interpretation.

TEACHING AND QUALITY CONTROL

There is no official or accredited training for the eight-week programme and the training on offer is very diverse. As a consequence, it is therefore difficult to implement quality control. As the head of an organisation of mindfulness coaches, I am trying to put things into perspective, more or less successfully I have to admit. The quality of classes and teachers in meditation can be problematic at times. Nowadays everyone can claim to be a therapist and I am unable at this stage to immediately give you a specific training programme that allows you to become a meditation teacher. As far as I am concerned, I use two informal criteria: profession and experience. When it comes to profession, I have seen too many depressed patients taking classes with teachers who had no medical or psychological background! Experience is paramount too, because you don't teach someone how to ski if you can hardly stand up on your own skis.

~

Chapter 9

Loving kindness meditation

~

'Few of us regret all the years dedicated to the
completion of a training or the mastery of an
important skill. So why bemoan the perseverance
needed to become a well-balanced and
compassionate human being?'

— MATTHIEU RICARD

One evening a Native American headman told his young grandson about the internal fight that takes place within all human beings.

'My dear grandson, in the heart of each human being there are two wolves constantly fighting each other. The first embodies Evil. He carries all our feelings of anger, jealousy, sadness, envy, arrogance and rancour... The other wolf is the embodiment of Kindness. He is full of joy, friendship, comfort, love, hope, quiet, understanding and compassion. Having thought it through, the grandson then asked, 'So which wolf wins in the end, grandpa?'

The old man simply replied, 'The wolf that you have fed most.'

My Canadian spouse descends from the Native American tribes of the First Nation Abenakis. The Abenaki were a deeply religious people who referred to the Earth as their "Grandmother" and considered that all animals and natural things, such as rocks and trees, had an individual spirit. My wife always insists that every day we are offered the possibility to choose between good and evil, recalling this lovely story to our kids of the two wolves that live together in our heart. Indeed, it so happens that you can feed the good wolf by taking up a specific form of meditation, the loving kindness meditation, which is the favourite form of my dear friend Matthieu.

Most meditation techniques, such as breathing meditation or mindfulness meditation, focus primarily on developing the mind and states of consciousness. Loving kindness meditation is also a technique that encourages the development of altruistic qualities, such as compassion, understanding, love and friendship. Loving kindness meditation aims to enhance those feelings towards both oneself and others – your loved ones, friends, enemies and strangers. This technique stems from the Buddhist tradition and is sometimes called 'metta' (meaning 'positive energy' and 'kindness towards others'). It is very versatile, however, and can be adapted and used by us all, whatever your personal persuasion or faith. Love is universal.

Loving kindness meditation is much more than the cultivation of benevolence. It helps us to be aware of others' needs and brings up true compassion towards others and the candid wish that their suffering is diminished. In order to attain such a deep feeling of compassion, one has to open up when meditating, so that one can feel what others around us feel too. Thus, loving kindness meditation focuses on altruism and self-abnegation. In other words, you learn how to care honestly for someone else and to love that person without any form of self-interest. It has been shown that this exercise goes far beyond the spiritual and studies have evidenced that loving kindness meditation could help healthcare professionals and teachers, who are often confronted with the pain of others, to ward off emotional burnout. The added value of meditation practices was also studied during the COVID-19 pandemic.[1]

Empathy-related stress and compassion in the lab

Empathy is a fundamental fact of life. It is a crucial quality needed to succeed in one's social life. Studies have shown how empathy greatly influences our decisions. In one of those,[2] participants were asked to show empathy towards a person who was receiving painful electric shocks. In fact, subjects were willing to receive electric shocks themselves and alleviate the suffering of the person in question. Empathy can, however, also cause stress, because when you experience the negative emotions of others it can lead you to feel emotionally overwhelmed, even hopeless, and therefore prone to forms of stress or burnout. Unfortunately, this is a phenomenon commonly observed among doctors, nurses and healthcare workers, and researchers at the Max Planck Institute have studied to what degree loving kindness meditation can remedy the negative effects of empathy.

Empathy and compassion are different mental states. The importance of compassion has been evidenced by Native Americans, Buddhists, psychologists and neurologists alike. My colleague and friend Tania Singer,[3] who is currently head of the Social Neuroscience Lab in Berlin and very active with Mind & Life Europe, defines empathy as being an affective state which resembles the affective state of another person and which appears at the moment when he or she observes that other, or is offered a representation of that situation by that other person. She describes compassion as the altruistic will to intervene in favour of a suffering person.

Let's take an example to illustrate the difference between empathy and compassion. Imagine that your travel buddy is scared stiff of flying. If, while sitting next to your friend, you are worried about him and share his fear, then it is empathy you are experiencing. And by the way, this may elicit

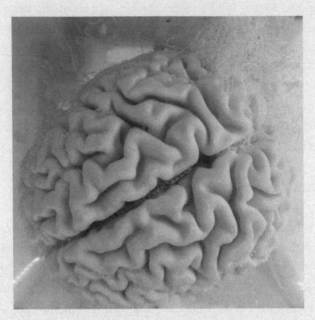

© Steven Laureys, in collaboration with Laurent Hermoye, who contributed the exact measurements of the brain, and Dr Fede Raimondo from our own team, who provided this beautiful 3D print-out.

'Meditation is brain fitness!'

The image above shows Matthieu Ricard's athletic brain, measured and printed out in three dimensions.

His brain is bigger than average, even when age, body weight, cranial circumference and gender have been factored in. As we grow older, our brain volume diminishes progressively. This process starts by the age of around 45 and, yes, I confess I have reached that stage! After the age of 85, a person will usually have lost about 10 per cent of their brain volume compared with the peak it reached at the age of 19, when the brain weighs approximately 1.45 kilos. Given all these parameters, we have established that Matthieu Ricard's brain is about 7 per cent bigger than the brain of an average man in his 70s, which in effect represents about 100 grams of additional brain mass. Rather impressive, isn't it? If we consider the specific brain structures on which meditation has a positive impact, such as the hippocampus, which is a key organ for our memory, then Matthieu is much better off than his peers as his brain presents an increased volume of 7 per cent. When I showed him the results, he laughed and joked, 'This way, I can store even more foolishness!' Several scientific studies have demonstrated that meditation exercises performed by the elderly can increase their brain volume and their brain connectivity (see page 52), as well as blood circulation in the brain. More importantly, elderly guinea pigs who pick up meditation report that they feel less stressed and enjoy a better quality of life. Several on-going studies are attempting to identify whether meditation and the networks it activates may be used as a complementary treatment for people at risk of dementia. As a preventive measure, I am already meditating... and I offered Matthieu Ricard the 3D print-out of his brain.[4]

similar feelings of anxiety and exhaustion. By contrast, if you are worried about him and hold his hand in order to assuage his fear, then it is compassion you are experiencing.

So what happened during the study? One group of participants followed a training programme in empathy while the other was trained in compassion. Both groups had to view videos of other people suffering. Empathic training increased negative affect as well as the engagement of brain areas associated with empathy, i.e., the anterior insula. By contrast, compassion training countered negative affect and reinforced positive affect by engaging the brain network that comprises the ventral striatum, the anterior cingulate cortex and the orbitofrontal cortex. We may therefore be in a position to conclude that compassion training could constitute a strategy to overcome the possible stress caused by empathy and therefore strengthen resilience.

How to practise loving kindness meditation
You do this by cultivating a feeling of unconditional love and compassion towards yourself and others, for example by repeating a benevolent phrase to yourself, such as, 'May all people on earth be content and find security.'

The fact that this elicits increased feelings of compassion and a greater capacity for benevolence towards others is not just idle talk. When we asked Matthieu to practise loving kindness meditation while lying in our lab's scanners, we could really see changes in his brain's activity.

The compassion brain network, which includes the insula and the anterior cingulate cortex and which is known to play a prime role in feelings such as love, is more active when this type of meditation is being practised. This points to a greater capacity to feel sympathy for others, without being overwhelmed by emotions. What's more, we also identified increased activity in the areas of the brain responsible for the capacity to put oneself in somebody else's place, to share their feelings and their take on things. In these studies researchers also found evidence that increased empathy not only has positive repercussions for those to whom the empathy was directly addressed, but also that it greatly benefited the person itself, although this is not what the researchers expected. Those who have greater compassion will suffer fewer negative feelings in general and also present with increased brain activity in the areas responsible for positive feelings. When you show kindness you are in fact happier. This is beneficial for all parties and may well be why the journalist described Matthieu as 'the happiest man in the world'.

Let's take an example. We can imagine (and I very frequently encounter this in my clinical practice) the extent to which it is difficult to have one's loved-one hospitalised for a serious brain injury after a traffic accident. Of course, this is terribly difficult both for the patient and the family. As a medical doctor, I have noticed that the family member who stays at the bedside to encourage and comfort their beloved suffers less from negative feelings such as anxiety and stress than the relative who nervously paces up and down the corridors of the hospital or intensive care unit. Feelings of love and comfort will not only help the patient but will also help the family to ward off emotional stress.

It is clear that no one expects you to walk in the steps of Matthieu Ricard or other experienced meditators. Loving kindness meditation requires a substantial amount of time and practice, and as far as I am concerned, it is not something obvious or that I feel I am a natural at. There is nothing wrong with having emotions. We are not robots and we can all experience resentment, anger or envy. We may also on occasion cry, bang our fists on the table or honk the horn without really thinking about it when caught in the chaos of a traffic jam. These things happen. To decide to work on it is a great – and a difficult – step, but I will help you by giving you a few tips and tricks for taking up this particular form of meditation, which is really for those who are at a more advanced level.

LOVING KINDNESS MEDITATION

Loving kindness meditation is synonymous with unconditional love. The objective during this type of meditation is to not discriminate between those who deserve your messages of love, happiness and empathy and those who don't. Your kindness, therefore, should be addressed not only to your loved ones and friends, but should also extend to all people around the world. What's more, you should practise loving kindness meditation without expecting anything in return. The deal is that you give pure, unconditional and altruistic love to all.

I can already hear your reservations. Surely this isn't very realistic? Well, obviously you aren't expected to feel love for Peter, Paul or John overnight. That is why loving kindness meditation generally unfolds over several stages. You need to learn how to awaken progressively warmer feelings in yourself. First, those warm feelings should be directed towards yourself, then towards your loved ones, then neutral people and those for whom it is more difficult to have those feelings, and, finally, to everyone around the world. To succeed you can repeat love messages while meditating. This is how to do it.

Seek out a place where you can sit comfortably and where you feel at ease, an environment, for instance, that triggers positive feelings in you. The starting point is to feel well, so make sure you choose a comfortable position that allows you to be as tranquil as possible. Once you have found that position, focus your attention on the middle of your ribcage and visualise your heart as the symbol of love.

Then take a deep breath in and a deep breath out, as if, in this meditation session, your breathing originated in your heart. As you inhale and exhale calmly, imagine that your mind and your heart are softening and warming to thoughts of love addressed to yourself. If you feel any mental block, or self-criticism and negative thoughts take over, refocus on the positive feelings and let other thoughts go. In order to feel this loving kindness you may want to choose from a variety of traditional love messages or you can formulate them in your own words, for instance, 'I am attentive and kind!'

Then think of the person who most invites such feelings of pure and unconditional love, of warm friendship, of love that expects nothing in return. The first person that springs to mind is usually a mentor, benefactor or an elderly person. It may be a parent, grandparent, teacher — someone who naturally commands respect and immediately inspires you to show solicitude. It can also be a baby you love, or your favourite pet, whatever works best for you.

Repeat the following sentence with this person in mind: 'May s/he be protected and be safe!' After having experienced strong feelings of unconditional love for this benefactor, you need to choose a good friend and repeat the sentence again. And remember to continue inhaling and exhaling from the bottom of your heart! Then select a neutral person who inspires neither positive nor negative feelings. Repeating that sentence will allow you to feel affectionate and benevolent towards yourself, to the benefit of your own wellbeing. Now select someone with whom you have a more fraught relationship, towards whom you feel resentment and harbour hostile feelings. Repeat the same sentence for this person. If you can't manage it, you may want to say, 'As far as I am concerned, I would like it that you...'

If you start feeling resentment towards the person again, turn your attention to the benefactor and let yourself be pervaded by a feeling of kind friendship. Then revert again to the person with whom you have a problematic relationship. Let the sentence permeate your body, mind and heart. After this difficult person, allow your loving kindness to reach out to all human beings.

'May all human beings be safe and sound, cheerful and happy... May all those who breathe be safe and sound, cheerful and happy... May all individuals be safe and sound, cheerful and happy... May all living humans...' May all these sentences be the source of inspiration for your loving kindness! Unleash your imagination on these sentences and may you touch the heart of all forms of life known on earth, unconditionally and inclusively. Concentrate on all beings until you attain a feeling of profound communion with all forms of life, with the whole of nature, with the whole universe.

~

TESTIMONIAL: JULES EVANS

**'Do I miss it when I don't do it? Yes, I think the day
is better with meditation and a good meditation is a
great start to the day.'**

~

*Jules Evans describes himself as a 'practical philosopher'. His mission is to
help people suffer less and flourish more. He researches ideas from different
eras and cultures, then tries them out in his own life, telling others about his
experiences through books – his most recent is* Breaking Open: Finding a
Way Through Spiritual Emergency *– courses, events and his website. I hope
you'll agree his story is fascinating.*

PSYCHEDELIC EXPERIMENTATION

So the story really starts with me and my friends as teenagers in London
taking a lot of psychedelic drugs and going raving. In some ways it was very
exciting, but we were way out of our depth. We were going into highly altered
states of consciousness when we were 16 or 17. I think we saw it as a rite
of passage — 'Hey, look how hard we are. We can get completely out of
our heads and we're fine' — but then some of my friends got into various
problems, from prison to overdosing, and I had a couple of bad LSD trips. I
had one bad LSD trip, but I kept on doing it and had another, and they were
very scary. I was very paranoid and I think what made these experiences
traumatising was that I didn't talk to anyone about them. I just didn't have
the emotional range or vocabulary, so I shut down.

As an English man you're trained to keep it all in and all through university — I
did English at Oxford — I was in a very bad way inside. The amazing thing was
my housemates didn't even know that I was going through this stuff. This is
Englishness! I knew something was wrong. I knew my personality had changed
a lot. I was much more neurotic, anxious, ruminating, than I had been before. I
was getting panic attacks. I didn't know what they were. I just knew that I was
having these excessive, weird, phobic reactions to ordinary social situations,
and I would dissociate, de-personalise. I now have the words for these things,

but right then I thought, 'Am I going mad? And is this permanent?' This was my big fear, at 19, on top of all my ambitions and social expectations: have I damaged myself permanently?

ATTEMPTS TO HEAL
When I was at Oxford I tried to heal. I don't remember being offered therapy by the university, but I did go to a meditation place. I'd read the Buddha at school, along with some Taoism and some Stoicism, and I thought, 'This sounds great.' I remember at 17 I thought, 'What I'll do is be really successful in the world, and then I'll renounce it all and become a monk.' I had this romantic idea of being a Taoist sage, so I went to a Shambhala meditation group and tried meditation there, but it was a bit off-putting. Every sentence began, 'As Chogyam Trungpa Rinpoche says...' so I found that a bit cultish.

Of course, at Oxford now they have a whole mindfulness for health and wellbeing programme and centre, but back then if you wanted to do meditation, you had to do advanced Buddhism, which was all about going beyond the self, and I wasn't in a good enough place to do that kind of advanced Buddhism. I was off-balance, so I would think, 'OK, if I meditate enough, I won't feel any pain and I'll be completely calm.' The calm would last for about an hour after I left the meditation place, and then one thing would trigger me and I'd be anxious again.

I managed to get through university and graduate, but then I had a kind of mini-breakdown when the social anxiety was really bad. I couldn't even get through a job interview without having a panic attack, but I did get a job as a financial journalist, and I was good at writing and thinking. That bit of my psyche wasn't damaged, it was my social skills and I found office life very hard. I was anxious, very sensitive, worried about getting on with the people in the office — I didn't get on with them very well — so by the age of 24 I was numb and really quite unwell, and had become a very different person to who I was at 17, much more introverted and isolated and neurotic.

NEAR-DEATH EXPERIENCE
Then I had this strange, near-death experience in Norway, where my family goes on holiday every year. On this particular trip, I skied through

a fence on a mountain and off the side of a cliff. I landed and broke my leg, two vertebrae and banged my head, but at the moment of impact I was immersed in a white light. I wasn't aware of my body, but just had this sense of being completely loved and well. I understood that there's something in you — one's 'soul' — that can't be damaged, even by death, and I had this great insight, a very deeply felt realisation, that it was my own beliefs, perpetuated by my need for approval, that was causing my suffering, not damaged neuro-chemistry, which is what I had feared. So that all happened in about two minutes, because the first thing I remember was coming to in my body and thinking, 'Oh, I've been in an accident.' I was quite rational. I thought I might be paralysed, so I tried to wiggle my toes and realised I could, and then, even though I couldn't actually speak, I knew that basically I'd be fine. I knew that something wonderful had happened to me.

For the next two months, even though I was extremely damaged physically, I felt extremely well. I felt spiritually regenerated and, you know, what luck, because that never happens to some people and I hadn't particularly earned it. I felt very reconnected to myself, able to relate to other people without anxiety, but then the old habits started to come back and to some extent the epiphany wore off, so I knew I needed some systematic ways to ingrain this insight, that it was my beliefs causing my suffering and that I could believe differently.

For some reason I knew that cognitive behavioural therapy [CBT] would do that, so I went along to a CBT support group for people who suffer from social anxiety. There was no therapist present, but one person had downloaded a CBT course called 'Overcoming Social Anxiety Step by Step', so this group followed the course and did the exercises, and after a couple of months I stopped having panic attacks. That got me interested in CBT, so I went to interview the people who invented it, Albert Ellis and Aaron Beck. They both told me they got it from Stoicism, which I'd read a bit about before, so through that I got into Greek philosophy and Stoicism in particular, and I wrote my first book on it. It was called *Philosophy for Life and Other Dangerous Situations* and it's really about how people use ancient Greek philosophies today for resilience and to flourish.

STOICISM AND BUDDHISM

So that's the first part of the story and it takes me to the age of about 35. At the time that book came out I was doing a lot of talks about Stoicism and Greek philosophy, and organising Stoic conferences, and Stoicism is similar to Buddhism as a cognitive theory of the emotions. If you compare quotes from Marcus Aurelius to the Buddha, they're very similar. Marcus talks about the well-guarded mind being like an inner citadel and the Buddha talks about the mind being like a well-thatched roof or a fortress. They both have this idea that what causes our emotions is our opinions or beliefs or thoughts. The first passage in the *Dhammapada* is, 'He abused me, he insulted me, he harmed me. People who think like that will have a harmful mind.' So it's this idea that suffering follows destructive thoughts like a cart follows a horse, and that's a very Stoic idea. The Stoic theory of the emotions is people are disturbed not by events, but by their opinions about events, and sometimes when I hear Buddhist talks, they could be talking about Stoicism.

Some even think that there's a direct link between India and Greece; that maybe Pythagoras, who's one of the fathers of Greek philosophy, went to India, because Pythagoras and Plato introduced the idea of reincarnation into Western culture. Certainly, Alexander the Great's army went to India and saw these Hindu fakirs and they called them *gymnosophists*, which means 'naked philosophers', so they recognised them as similar to their own Greek philosophers.

In both Greek philosophy and Buddhism there's this idea of a kind of scepticism; that the desire for over-certainty can cause you suffering; that because we're afraid of uncertainty, we very much hold on to beliefs. Both Buddhism and to some extent Greek philosophies say, 'Sometimes it's your beliefs that are causing you suffering, so just try being OK with uncertainty.' Rather than saying, 'I know that I could never do this or this person hates me, well, who knows? Maybe, maybe not.' So being a little wary of one's automatic opinions and assumptions is very useful.

So Stoicism and Greek philosophy really helped me and I became a Stoic. I even got a Stoic tattoo on my arm, but after a few years of Stoicism I began to feel it missed some things out. It was very rational. It says that the way to flourishing is rationality and it also has a rather unusual relation to emotions, so you're trying to transcend all negative emotions to achieve the state of *apatheia*, which is really 'beyond emotion'. That's the goal, but what that can mean in practice is you have trainee Stoics denying their emotions, shutting down instead and not being honest with themselves.

Stoicism also says you should become free of all attachments and aversions, a bit like Buddhism, but if you are a traumatised young man whose attachment style is 'anxious avoidant', then actually what you need to do is learn how to relate to others, how to be dependent on others and how to make attachments. So if you're traumatised Stoicism can be helpful, but it can also be maladaptive, because it's very individualistic and self-reliant, and I recognised that I needed to try and gain the capacity to make attachments.

ECSTATIC EXPERIENCES

So I then looked for other ways to heal more deeply and to get in touch with that kind of white light experience, because near-death experiences are definitely wonderful, but you're also left with a sense of longing. What was that place? How do I get back to it? So in my second book, *The Art of Losing Control*, I looked at how people find ecstatic experiences in Western culture, and when they're good for us and when they're bad for us. That meant looking at everything from ecstatic Christianity — I joined the Church for a year, I became a Christian, although I didn't get a tattoo that time — to psychedelics — I looked at the new psychedelic research and eventually tried psychedelics again — to the arts and music and literature. In that book there was a chapter on contemplation and that led me deeper into Buddhism again.

I'd never really walked away from Buddhism, but I must have been 37 or 38 and for the first time I went to do a meditation retreat at the Vipassana Centre in Sweden, and it was so full on. You go from having meditated for 30 minutes max to meditating for 10 hours a day for 10 days. It's incredibly intense. I found it very physically painful, because I wasn't used to crossing my legs for that long, but you realise that your attention can shift hugely in its quality in that time and you end up being able to concentrate on your breathing or just your nostrils for an hour at a time. Vipassana's teaching is that both painful and pleasurable experiences, including ecstasy, are just experiences, they are temporary, and that was very useful advice for that book. What was also useful about Vipassana was realising that philosophy needs to be somatic. You learn to examine, for example, the transience of things at the level of physical sensations; you learn to practise equanimity in the face of physical suffering or physical euphoria. So in that sense it was deeper than CBT or Stoicism, because it was so about physical awareness.

One of my issues with Stoicism was it was so individualist, so I tried to engage with Buddhist sanghas, communities, because I recognise the importance of community, but that isn't easy. Take a Vipassana community, for instance — you go there, it's a silent retreat and then you leave. There's no church to Vipassana. It's very modern, secularised, individualised. I then tried to join the Rigpa. That's another community, but, guess what, the head of Rigpa turned out to be a sex pest and then a fraud. I'm talking about Sogyal Rinpoche, whose book, *The Tibetan Book of Living and Dying*, was one of my favourite books as a teenager. So then I joined the London Buddhist Centre. It's called Triratna and, guess what, the founder of that turned out to be a sex pest. Or you could join Shambhala, and guess what, the founder of that turns out to be a sex pest. So it's challenging to find communities that don't have skeletons in the past. What I've come to accept is that every community has a skeleton in the past and what matters more is the quality of the people in there now and the quality of their relationships.

BUDDHISM AND ME

When I was 13, I refused to be confirmed, apparently because I said, 'I'm a Buddhist.' I haven't taken the vows, but yes, I'm a Buddhist. I've got a Stoic tattoo and I did commit my life to Jesus, but Buddhism has stayed with me longer than any other philosophy. Buddhism is very important to me and the *dharma* is very important to me. It's good to have goals in life and they say that the first level of attainment in Buddhism is 'stream entry', so in the years I have left I would like to try to attain stream entry as a goal.

I meditate every morning, five out of seven days a week. Sometimes if I'm very hungover or have had a bad night's sleep I might not. I wake up, check my phone, read the internet for about 30 minutes and then meditate. I have a meditation mat and I have worked out how to sit comfortably, because my legs and back are still not great after that injury, so I put two cushions underneath and tuck my legs under me. Then I use a meditation timer on my phone, so I will do it for maybe 20 minutes, maybe 30 minutes. On the whole,

I will either do mindfulness of breath, just counting my breath, or sometimes slow breath if I'm a bit anxious, which is when I breathe in for five seconds, then breathe out for seven seconds. That's a very helpful technique for me. It's very helpful when I'm playing tennis as well. If I lose my temper during tennis, I do five-seven breathing and it makes a massive difference. It's very good for regulating emotion.

Do I miss it when I don't do it? Yes, I think the day is better with meditation and a good meditation is a great start to the day. It reduces the 'noise' and gives me a bit of space to relate to my thoughts. I've learned to be more aware of what's going on in my body and what I am feeling. If you're quite an intellectual, bookish person, you can sometimes be quite detached from what you're feeling and what's happening in your body, so it can be useful to go, 'OK, I'm feeling angry at the moment' or 'I'm feeling sad.'

I also appreciate in Buddhism the idea of meditating on the impermanence of the body. It's not much talked about as a practice or taught, but I do think that it's useful to consider that you're going to die, so you can rehearse that. There's also this the sense that your body is not you. Spirituality has become wellness in Western culture and wellness is very much the cult of the beautiful body, but massively over-identifying with your body can be a recipe for suffering. I find it helpful to imagine that we have been countless people and bodies over countless lives, so there's no need to get particularly hung up on any one body or personality.

I personally think you can use Buddhist practices for wellbeing. In some ways that's not Buddhism, but that's totally fine. Likewise, you can use Stoic practices for wellbeing and not be a stoic, and I don't have any problem with that. Buddhism seems to me to depend on certain supernatural beliefs, at least the belief in reincarnation and karma, but I'm not a fundamentalist — whatever helps people when they're suffering.

~

Chapter 10

Mindfulness for health workers, athletes, students and inmates

~

'Perhaps this is why it is said that great poetry is born in silence. Great music and art are said to arise from the quiet depths of the unconscious, and true expressions of love are said to come from a source which lies beneath words and thoughts. So it is with the greatest efforts in sports; they come when the mind is as still as a glass lake.'

— W. TIMOTHY GALLWEY, author

Work occupies a great deal of our time and there is nothing wrong with that per se. Work can sometimes give meaning to your life. Unfortunately, many people complain about their workload and the stress that comes with it. No company is spared. And too much stress makes people unhappy and therefore it may be a factor in high levels of health-related absenteeism or even cause a high risk of professional exhaustion. For instance, in the Netherlands about 14 per cent of workers complain that they are suffering from burnout. A study carried out by the Catholic University of Leuven[1] with the medical and nursing staff of Belgian hospitals has shown that 40 per cent of them suffer from emotional exhaustion. This percentage reaches upto 50 per cent in the UK, 60 per cent in the USA and 80 per cent in Singapore[2]!

As medical workers, we practise in a high-risk profession, risks that are discussed too little and for which no preventive measures have been implemented. What's more, several studies[3] have shown that as a doctor I run a 70 per cent increased risk of dying by suicide than other men of my age. Among female doctors this risk increases by 250 to 400 per cent! In France, one doctor in two suffers from burnout. At least that appears to be the staggering conclusion of a recently published study based on the testimony of some 15,000 practitioners working in hospitals or outpatient care, as well as 37 other scientific studies carried out in various French hospitals between 2000 and 2017.[4] That's why I am passionate about supporting the Belgian platform doctors4doctors.be, an initiative taken by medics themselves and which offers mindfulness-based compassionate living (MBCL) programmes, the latter emphasising training in compassion and self-compassion for doctors suffering from mental exhaustion. In Belgium, as elsewhere, the exhaustion suffered by medical staff is very alarming and it is shocking that no structural measures have been implemented by way of prevention. This is also why I have co-founded the Mind Care International Foundation – a non-profit organisation whose mission it is to take care of the mind – in both health and disease, for patients and care-givers alike.

Chronic stress not only leads to burnout, but also sabotages key professional skills: close collaboration, creative research solutions and judicious decision-making. Excessive stress should therefore be combatted. Initiatives to take the pressure off should be implemented by offering programmes of psychological support or of mindfulness, or by encouraging workers to take up regular physical exercise. I am particularly proud of all the organisations that foster the practice of meditation and sport, because these activities allow their staff to efficiently reduce stress.

But how does the practice of mindfulness pay off at work? In the previous chapters, we mentioned several studies that evidenced how meditation improves stress symptoms and boosts concentration. A recent analysis of the scientific literature specifically addressing the question of mindfulness at work concludes that mindfulness has a positive influence on businesses. Just like Matthieu, I don't agree with the detractors of meditation in the workplace who argue that it is a cynical calculation by employers to increase productivity.

Employees who take up training in mindfulness have reported increased wellbeing, as well as enhanced relationships and improvements in their judgements and general capacity to work. Furthermore, mindfulness has also been linked with better metacognition, which is our faculty to observe and take stock of our thoughts and feelings, and the fact that the way we think things look doesn't necessarily reflect 'reality' or 'the truth'. The more this faculty is developed, the better the person is equipped to make conscious choices, rather than be the victim of automatic reactions.

There is also another interesting link between mindfulness and decision-making skills. Have you heard of the global cost analysis principle? No? You should be familiar with it, because it's the reason why people don't dare to end a relationship that doesn't work. It is also what causes people to watch a bad film until the end because, supposedly, 'They have seen more than half of it.' And, finally, it's why investors don't sell stocks that nevertheless continue to lose value. This global cost analysis is what drives us to persist in something, because we have already invested time or money in it. A study carried out by the INSEAD Business School[5] brought to light that 15 minutes of mindfulness a day contributes to reducing this behavioural tendency and therefore enables people to make more astute decisions. To test this, participants were invited to imagine they were entrepreneurs who had just bought an expensive printing press. Were they prepared to spend an extra 10,000 dollars to purchase a new automated press that would allow the business to work much more efficiently? Before the question was put to them, participants were split into two groups. The first group had to do mindfulness exercises every 15 minutes, whereas the second group simply had to let their thoughts 'stray'. In the first group, about eight out of 10 participants chose to buy the new press, against four out of 10 in the control group.

Bolstered by promising studies and different commercial stakeholders, meditation has made its first steps within the business world. In Zuidas, one of the main financial districts of Amsterdam, mindfulness is booming. In Belgium, Colruyt, the chain of retail stores, has also invested in mental health training programmes for its managers and in-store employees, with Jef Colruyt, the managing director, setting the trend. For the first time in France, and following the British initiative of 2004 that offered meditation sessions to MPs, French parliamentarians and their teams took part in a presentation on mindfulness given by psychiatrist Christophe André.

Should we start investing massively in mindfulness? Anne Speckens, psychiatry professor at Radboud University in the Netherlands, finds businesses' enthusiasm for mindfulness very understandable: 'We spend a substantial part of our time at work being submitted to an ever-growing number of pressures. If we are in a position to teach people to reflect on what they feel and think, and how they deal with events, then mindfulness surely can only have a positive effect on healthcare workers, athletes and sports people, students and inmates, as well as the general work environment. And by the same token, also on the final product.' But there is also a real danger that businesses resort to mindfulness with the sole purpose of boosting their revenues, rather than to improving the wellbeing of their employees. Dr Speckens therefore underscores how important it is to 'double-check the credentials of those who do the training and what promises are being made' when one wishes to use mindfulness as an employee or employer.

Personally, I am a firm believer in healthy, pleasant and empowering workplaces, and I also think that, alongside offering formal meditation training, it is also very useful to foster a mindfulness culture that encourages informal meditation.[6] One can easily go for a brief walk between tasks and avoid multitasking, giving one's full attention to all tasks and completing them one by one.

Mindfulness welcomed with open arms in Silicon Valley and Wall Street

A few years back, meditation was still associated with an alternative lifestyle, if not simply taboo. It was fashionable among a small circle of maverick hippies, but it was certainly not the done thing among managers and entrepreneurs, who need to have both their feet on the ground. But the times are over when mindfulness belonged exclusively to those who espoused 'peace and love'. Just look at what is happening in California or New York, two places that serve as the barometer for new cultural or medical trends. In Silicon Valley, in the San Francisco Bay area, numerous small start-ups as well as some of the most powerful technology businesses in the world have been won over by meditation and mindfulness. And the same goes for the big bosses in Wall Street, who consider meditation to be their new caffeine. Even the American Army uses mindfulness as mental training for its soldiers and it has now become part of their curriculum, although these dubious uses of meditation are often focused solely on profit, and strip meditation from its spiritual dimension and the exercises of empathy, compassion and altruism it should entail.

Many business leaders share their meditation habits with their employees, as well as the rest of the world. Jeff Weiner, CEO of LinkedIn, uses a different meditation exercise offered by the Headspace app every day and regularly tweets about the scientifically proven advantages of meditation. As far as he is concerned, these meditation exercises help him define the long-term strategy and objectives of his company. The head of Twitter, Jack Dorsey, has been using Vipassana meditation for over 20 years and recently gave himself a silent retreat in Myanmar (formerly Burma) for his birthday. This very rich entrepreneur meditated for 17 hours every day. He slept in a tiny and very austere cell on a bed with no mattress. Media, reading, writing, conversation and even visual contact were strictly forbidden. After the retreat he listened to the album *Damn* by Kendrick Lamar, and he explained that, as was the case after each retreat, it made for a unique experience, because he perceived each note as an individual event. As far as I'm concerned, my favorite meditation music is *The Anatomy Of Doubt* by piano composer Jef Martens. What is yours?

Steve Jobs, legendary creator of Apple, also had a predilection for yoga and meditation well before he became one of the most influential CEOs of his generation. According to him, meditation allowed him to feel less stressed, to think more coherently and be more creative. He acknowledged that a great number of his bold professional decisions were influenced by the fact that he trained his mind in meditation. Nowadays Apple has to do without Steve Jobs, but employees still have the chance to meditate and do mindfulness sessions.

Steve Jobs, legendary creator of Apple, also had a predilection for yoga and meditation well before he became one of the most influential CEOs of his generation.

At Google, another giant technology company, staff are offered training programmes that all bear alluring titles, such as Neural Self-Hacking, Managing your Energy etc. Google has even built a life-size labyrinth so that staff can do walking meditation and since Zen monk Thich Nhat Hanh came to visit the company, mindfulness pauses with absolute silence are being held at noon every day. The most impressive programme, however, is one entitled Search Inside Yourself. Initially it was just a low-key initiative launched by Google engineer Chade-Meng Tan, but it rapidly grew into a large-scale training programme taken by thousands of people.

Originally Chade-Meng wanted to help his colleagues 'unload their mental luggage and put them in a position where they can face each new situation being fully present mentally.' Meanwhile, his project has become a fully fledged independent programme that is on offer to employees around the world, notably in companies such as Ford and Trivago. Karen May, vice-CEO at Google, sticks to her rule of a single mindfulness breath before she enters a board meeting and, I admit, I try to follow her rule! You may deem this either banal or crazy, but as I have already explained, conscious and calm breathing gives a moment of mental and physical peace and engages the parasympathetic nervous system, which in turn has a soothing effect on the body and the brain. As Matthieu has very compellingly observed, Silicon Valley is not a paragon of humanism or altruism, but the healthy approaches such as the one presented by Chade-Meng are nevertheless heart-warming.

Yet the technology companies' infatuation with mindfulness should not come as a real surprise. High-tech activities rest on logical and well-under-pinned decisions. These businesses therefore rely on collaborators who do not merely take dictation from their monkey mind, but instead allow their prefrontal cortex to dominate. And meditation has the capacity to encourage just that... Currently, our team is studying the brain and mindset of entre-preneurs, using international surveys and brain-imaging measures aimed at understanding and promoting more compassionate entrepreneurship. Please see the testimony of Wouter Torfs on page 188–92 for more on this.

Learning to meditate at school

Is mindfulness useful in educational settings? More and more schools are concerned with the mental wellbeing of their students and are foregrounding mindfulness sessions in the curriculum. My colleague Filip Raes, psychology professor at the University of Leuven in Belgium, and his team undertook to assess the merits of this growing enthusiasm and studied the effects of mindful-ness on teenagers. To find out, they carried out a study in nine schools with 600 pupils. One group received mindfulness training, while the other just followed the classical curriculum. Adolescents represent an interesting study popula-tion, because their brains, besides being more malleable and therefore more sensitive to stress and physical ailments, also absorb new knowledge faster.

What were the results? Let's start with the good news: in the mindful-ness group, symptoms of stress, anxiety and depression decreased, with no variation between genders or between school levels. However, in the absence of control studies on meditation in schools, researchers advise against spending large budgets on expensive mindfulness programmes. Fortunately, other initiatives have been launched. Myriad,[7] a project led by the University of Oxford in the UK, is rather promising, for instance. It spans five years and involves over 5000 students.

These researchers also reckon that, 'There is less evidence for the benefits that mindfulness has in an educational setting than in a clinical setting.' They have indicated, however, that meditation and mindfulness can no doubt be useful tools, but insist that neither can resolve all student issues. In line with my friend, the French philosopher and avid meditator Fabrice Midal,[8] I believe that meditation should not be used as a means to 'keep quiet' the young, students or employees, but rather as a technique that allows them to develop their own identity, assertiveness, and to learn to be emotionally more attentive in their interactions with others.

Other studies on meditation in educational settings have also been carried out in the United States. The positive conclusions of Professor Raes and his team were echoed in the results of a study carried out in the schools of an underprivileged and difficult neighbourhood in Baltimore, where the young are constantly confronted with poverty, violence and drug addiction. Students aged between six and 18, and born into low-income families, followed the MBSR mindfulness programme. So what were the results of this study? Most of the students displayed a decreased level of negative emotions, stress, depression and hostility towards themselves... In an ongoing study (in collaboration with Professor Lieven Annemans from the University of Ghent) we are currently assessing the effect of meditation in over 600 Flemish students. We are measuring its effect on their psychological wellbeing, pro-social behavior and learning performance.

Meditating behind bars

Prison inmates suffer more from physical and mental ailments than the rest of the population. They will have the tendency to rehash the dark events they experienced and life behind bars is often a source of stress. As we now know, stress can be really harmful to your mental and physical health. Can meditation and mindfulness help all these people who are in prison? Several studies seem to be very promising on this topic, and recommend yoga and mindfulness programmes in prisons.[9]

My dear friend Reginald Deschepper, retired Professor at the University of Brussels, and his collaborators, of which I am one, are currently working on a unique study. During six weeks inmates are being asked to do meditation exercises. The aim is to evaluate whether these exercises are beneficial health-wise. We are monitoring various parameters in this study. In particular, we are looking at the variability of the inmates' heart rate, because low heartbeat variability is associated with various underlying health issues. We are also measuring the length of inmates' telomeres, because as we have seen in previous chapters, telomeres shorten with age and meditation can delay this process.

Matthieu showed me a remarkable experiment carried out in India on how meditation has been used to facilitate the rehabilitation of inmates held at the prison in Tihar, a prison notorious for its extreme harshness.[10] The film made about it has inspired other correctional institutions, such as the North Rehabilitation Facility in Seattle, to use meditation and the Vipassana technique in particular by way of rehabilitation.

Matthieu also told me the story of Fleet Maull, an American sentenced to 25 years in prison for a drugs offence in 1985:[11] 'It was really a hellish environment: a sort of steel chamber inside a concrete flat-roofed building. There were no windows, no ventilation, no place where you could go for a small walk. These cells were overcrowded and incredibly hot. Noise was unrelenting; it was just anarchy. Inmates were fighting and yelling. Four or five televisions were on at the same time 24/7. That is when I started to sit down and meditate for the first time every day. I ended up meditating four to five hours per day on the upper bunk in a cell that was originally meant for two people. Sweat dropped down my face and into my eyes. In the beginning it was really hard, but I simply persevered.' After eight years of detention, Maull declared that this whole experience convinced him of 'the double truth of spiritual practice linked to the power of compassion and the illusionary reality of the "self",' specifying that this was not a Romantic idea, but his 'own direct experience'.

One day he received a message informing him that the health of a hospitalised inmate with whom he had worked had suddenly deteriorated. During the following five days, in between intensive sessions of meditation, he stayed for hours at the bedside of the inmate, helping him through his last hours: 'He had difficulties breathing and was vomiting blood; I was helping him to stay clean... Since those days I have often felt an immense sense of freedom and great joy. A kind of joy that transcends all circumstances, because it doesn't have an external cause and nothing in this prison could have nurtured it. It boosted a heightened confidence in my practice: I experienced something indestructible in the face of the spectacle of suffering and depression that is far beyond what is normally tolerable.' This story poignantly illustrates how happiness depends on our inner state. Otherwise, such serenity and sense of plenitude would have been inconceivable in such circumstances.

Meditation and sports performance

Score a three-point field goal during the very last seconds of a match under the eyes of millions of spectators, run the decisive 1500 metres after nine exhausting trials to know whether or not you are on the podium... Because during a competition, a mere split-second lapse of attention can be the difference. It can make you win or lose, send you to the locker room or raise you to the podium, make you rich or lead to your sponsors dropping you. Yet it is a fact that several studies have shown that mindfulness helps athletes to increase performance, better deal with stress and to fight burnout.[12]

Top athletes have lots to teach us about how to perform under pressure and therefore on the influence of stress, the importance of focus and mental resilience. 'Elite' athletes are physically and technically all as good as each other. Just look at the case of tennis. It is not unheard of that a tennis player ranked 70th in the world league table beats one of the top 10 players because he feels 'invincible' that day.

It should not come as a surprise either that many top athletes use mindfulness and meditation. Tennis champion Novak Djokovic practises meditation on a daily basis as a means to better manage his stress and anxiety. He also does it to fulfil his need for quiet and maximise his state of mind. Moreover, Djokovic believes that breathing is the one most important thing for a human being. 'You need to be able to control it in order to face up to the pressure of stressful situations,' he argues.

In his book *Serve to Win*,[13] he gives several concrete examples of how mindfulness has helped him in his world-class achievements. 'After a few sessions of mindfulness meditation, my brain works better. It is as simple as that. Even when I am not meditating. I used to be petrified when I made a mistake and I was convinced I would never join the top tier players like Federer.' I should remind you here that in 2019 he won the Wimbledon men's single finals against his idol, Federer, in an epic match now considered to have made history. 'Nowadays, I still go through moments of doubt when I fail a service or a backhand stroke, but I know how to handle them. I recognise negative thoughts. I let them go so that I can focus on the present moment. Focusing my attention helps me to manage pains and emotions which in turn helps me to focus on what really matters. It helps me shut up the little internal voice.'

During a game pause at the NBA finals of 2012, LeBron James started to breathe calmly, eyes closed, in front of millions of spectators. The American basketball superstar not only meditates during crucial moments, but also every morning for 15 minutes in the quiet of his house. He uses the Calm app to guide him through his session. Other NBA legends such as Michael Jordan also meditate regularly, as did the late Kobe Bryant.

'A meditation session prepares me for the whole day. When I don't meditate in the morning, I have the impression I am late with everything that is happening around me. Meditation gives me the impression that I'm in control of what is happening to me,' comments Phil Jackson, one of the NBA coaches who boasts the greatest numbers of awards, and who has introduced mindfulness sessions to his training to strengthen the mental capacity of his players. He tried out several techniques, teaching them to meditate formally, introducing full days of silence and having the team play in near darkness.

Football icon Lionel Messi has also invested in his mental health and is another passionate advocate for meditation. On top of that, he takes care of his nutritional health and is a vegetarian. When you watch his magnificent penalties, he really seems to know how to focus his attention mindfully! Andy Puddicombe, former Buddhist monk and co-founder of Headspace, believes that, 'Meditating is about finding a balance between effortless relaxation and applied focus.' Lionel Messi provides an excellent example of such balance. The Headspace digital platform, which offers guided meditation sessions, has enlisted several Premier League footballers as clients. Andy Puddicombe also believes that, 'Meditation fosters spatial awareness skills, mental stamina and pain management. Muscles develop and strengthen during rest not during training. Therefore, factoring in adequate rest time is crucial.' According to him, meditating for 10 minutes after a football match allows players to assuage muscular pain. Researchers at the University Hospital of Oslo in Norway observed that sportspeople who practise meditation after intensive training manage to reduce the production of lactic acid, a by-product of anaerobic exercise that induces pain, and to restore their levels of physical wellbeing more quickly. In the recuperation tests carried out on athletes divided into several groups, researchers observed that the level of lactic acid in the blood was lower among the men who had done meditation sessions than among those in the control group.[14]

The list of sportspeople who consider meditation to be a crucial element of their training is very long. Raymond van Barneveld, one of the most successful darts players in history, has learnt to improve his capacity to focus thanks to his Zen master. The world-champion has claimed that he now feels 'wholly serene' during a competition, whereas in the past he would have been totally paralysed by stress. Studies have indeed evidenced that mindfulness improves performance in precision sport like darts or shooting.[15] Other examples include European marathon champion Koen Naert, who has been meditating for six years. Or Tom Brady, the most talented quarterback player in the history of American football, a meditation devotee, who recently posted the following on his Instagram account: 'It is when the mind is as still as a glass lake that the greatest sports effort can occur.'

Talking about extraordinary physical performances and frozen lakes, it is impossible not to mention the name of Wim Hof. This Dutchman, nicknamed the Ice Man, holds many Guinness world records. He spent more than six hours in a tub filled with ice and ran a marathon in the Sahara without drinking any water, but he doesn't put his achievements down to extraordinary talent or an iron will. According to him, everyone is capable of doing what he has done. The key, he claims, lies in his method, which combines breathing techniques, exposure to cold and meditation.

But does it really work? What do our research colleagues say about the influence of mindfulness on sports performance? One of the first to have studied this possible link is Jon Kabat-Zinn, the father of mindfulness-based stress reduction (MBSR). His study group was made up of rowers who had won Olympic medals. The athletes indicated that mindfulness improved their capacity to focus and relax, while decreasing the effects of pain and negative thought.[16]

But can this enhancement of sports performance thanks to meditation also be observed in the brain? A research team in San Diego looked into this in collaboration with the national BMX team – an extreme cycling sport that is physical, technical and quite spectacular. The results of the study showed increased neural activity when the athletes anticipated their performance, as well as during intense physical activity. The results also evidenced a greater capacity to optimise performance under extreme stress.[17]

An overarching analysis of the results of 26 studies on the link between mindfulness and sports performance[18] seems to foreground empirical arguments, stating, 'Mindfulness is a relevant characteristic of performance when it comes to sport' and that mindfulness can be useful for athletes. Let's quote, for instance, improved focus, concentration, acceptance, feeling in control, awareness of physical sensation and the diminishing of anxiety and stress. This analysis underlines again the need for more highly qualitative studies and for more thorough evaluation. In our lab we are now studying the activity of the mind and brain in endurance runners who are getting 'in the zone' or experience 'flow'. We are comparing how this mental state – in which one is fully immersed in a feeling of energised focus, full involvement, and enjoyment of the process of the activity – compares to mindfulness and meditation.[19]

TESTIMONIAL: THOMAS VAN DER PLAETSEN

'Meditation is a powerful tool that helps me
to develop and improve.'

~

Mindfulness has been the defining element in the life of Thomas Van der Plaetsen, decathlete and European champion. His story, which has been marked by spectacular reversals and heroic comebacks, is just like a movie. For him, mindfulness is essentially the awareness of his inner world, as it helps him to better grasp his emotions and thoughts. Mindfulness progressively found a home in his life until it settled in permanently. It gave him the resilience necessary to cope when he was diagnosed with cancer and had to undergo treatment. Thomas is one of those men who has built their own destiny and he learnt to apply mindfulness on an everyday basis without formal training, but finding inspiration in the books he read and the people he has around him.

MY MEDITATIVE QUEST

As a child, I often saw my parents meditating or doing yoga. My father was a neuropsychiatrist who worked at the hospital, but he would also have patient consultations at home. Throughout his career, religion and meditation mattered greatly to him and he also studied the brains of a number of meditation practitioners. This is how mindfulness and spirituality entered my life. There was no taboo at home regarding these matters. But because I was diagnosed with ADHD as child, contemplative meditation was not for me.

After my father's death in 2011, I felt lost. It was a difficult period of my life. I was hardly 20, I lacked self-confidence and I even had to fight an aggressive form of measles! At the same time, I did win a gold medal at the European Athletics U23 Championships, but I still felt that emotionally I was all over the place. I then decided to take matters into my own hands and went in search of answers to the questions that I had about myself and that were haunting me. My quest for spirituality and the great existential questions I had led me to read several books on meditation and Buddhism, in particular, *Happiness: A Guide to Developing Life's Most Important Skill* by Matthieu Ricard.

I love trying out new things. That's also true when it comes to sport, as I regularly try out new strategies that may help me to improve. That's why I experimented with meditation. In the beginning my sessions were rather simple. I had a book that told me how to do it and I started very slowly with one session a day. As a top athlete, I was already used to focusing on my breathing. I would breathe calmly for 10 to 15 minutes, allowing my thoughts to wander freely. I also successfully tried out Headspace for a short while, but after two months I found that those guided sessions slowed me down. With app sessions, everything is set up in advance, and I like surprises and have the propensity to go with the flow. With Headspace, after a number of sessions, you need to pass levels and tests. For me that makes it more like a video game!

MY MEDITATION EPIPHANY

After a few years, my practice took another turn; it became a lifestyle. I dropped conscious meditation and instead of meditating at certain times of the day, my days themselves became more meditative. I started to keep track of what I felt inside me throughout the day. From then on, my warm-ups would always start with being mindfully aware of the moment and with focusing on my inner self. Just like yoga, my warm-up session constituted a moment of meditation. Most of the time that is easy enough, given that I train by myself. During the day I also tried to find moments of peace and quiet. On the train for instance, I would tend to leave my smartphone in my bag more and more often. Mindfulness became a sort of compass that guided me to the origins of my thoughts and emotions. This daily training has made me more aware of the processes unfolding around me. Over time, specific exercises gave way to a mode of being.

That also translates into my relationships, in particular when conflicts arise. I believe it is important to identify any hostility resulting from a misunderstanding or misconception. This is how mindfulness has become a powerful tool to help me develop and improve.

Meditation has had a positive influence on me both as a man and as an athlete. I used to let myself be overwhelmed by a number of frustrations when I was training and this impacted my performance negatively. Upon reflection, I told myself that I could not continue to harm my development by reacting badly. Thanks to meditation I came to understand that a great number of negative feelings came from my lack of self-confidence and poor self-image. This realisation was a first step, but changing things was easier said than done. When a negative thought popped up, I couldn't manage to push it back. That is when I started training.

FASHION FADS AND SMOOTHIES

Meditation has clearly become a fashion. Some people meditate twice a day, but still continue to live exactly the same life. Some people don't dare to confront their issues and will just do with some heart balm: that's the illness of the century. When overweight, some people will just grab a vegetable smoothie rather than calling into question their diet and their sedentary lifestyle. Even the expression 'mindfulness meditation' has progressively become loaded with a certain connotation that harms its credibility. That's why I have decided not to use the expression anymore when I speak at conferences, because I have noticed the concept is misunderstood. Instead I talk about 'awareness', which means the same, in my view.

FALSE ACCUSATIONS AND CANCER

On 30 September 2014 I received a letter from the doping control authorities that I had tested positive for HCG hormone, an illegal product that enhances performance. 'That's it, my career is over!' I thought. I had no idea how the product had ended up in my blood, because I had not done any doping. Clinical examination confirmed on 30 October what I had found after a quick Google search: the HCG hormone was a marker of testicular cancer and I was gravely ill. Meanwhile, the press had already trashed my name and made me into yet another doped athlete. It was totally outlandish!

After my operation, I had chemo for a month. Mental training came in handy again at that moment. I decided quickly not to complicate the matter further and that my priority was to cope with uncertainty. My feeling was that, since I had no control over my future, I had better just accept it. Luckily, when I was diagnosed my mental training was already well advanced. Without the mindfulness and meditation I already had under my belt, I would not have been able to accept the cancer diagnosis that positively. If this had happened when I was 20, it would have been a totally different story.

I never really meditated formally during the treatment, but I was aware of all the thoughts that were going through my mind. What mattered most was that I was able to regulate my emotional world, and to control my pain and fatigue. I felt that I was stronger thanks to my mental training and that my negative thoughts failed to make me waver. A number of things didn't leave any precise memories. Chemotherapy was rather taxing, it weakened me mentally, but I didn't fight against the injustice of the situation.

BACK ON TRACK – AND SCEPTICISM ABOUT MINDFULNESS

As a well-known athlete, I ended up in the limelight while I underwent chemo, whereas most cancer patients heroically fight the illness without any attention. That's how the idea of creating Back on Track came to me. It is a fund that gives support and encouragement to cancer patients. We offer them a programme, including a range of physical exercises, and psychological and social support. We recently added mindfulness workshops. When participants first heard of it, they weren't overwhelmingly enthusiasm and couldn't really see the use of it. Later on, several admitted that they had really benefited from these sessions. Personally, I have never been sceptical about spirituality. When I read Matthieu's book on meditation, for instance, I never felt the need to criticise it.

PHILOSOPHY AND RELIGION

I consider myself a believer, but I am not convinced by any religion in particular. Meditation is also part of my religious quest. My parents passed on to me their Christian culture and values, from which I drew precious principles. I also find Buddhism very interesting. The concepts professed by Buddha are particularly clear and practical. They allow us to understand the role of our thoughts and emotions, and how to manage them. For instance, if you get cross with someone, the insidious venom of your thoughts is within you, not the other person. Over time, I developed my own philosophy. The Stoic philosophers, Seneca and Marcus Aurelius, are important sources of inspiration for me. They also emphasise introspection and the acceptance of the external world.

PAIN AND MIND GAMES

As a sportsman you are constantly confronted with pain. This is why I have massages three times a week with a physiotherapist. Half of these sessions are painful. Lying down on the table, I will consciously manage my pain. It has almost become a game in which I am trying to see how I can face these painful sensations. I have two tactics. The first consists of not thinking about it at all. I empty my inner self, I let all sensations come as they are and try to react as little as possible. The second tactic consists of focusing entirely on the pain. Just as with emotions, few of the painful sensations remain when you give them your full attention. I have been playing this mind game for a long time. Even in everyday life. If I have an itch, for instance, I try and see how long I can refrain from scratching it.

Informal meditation has become a habit, is now part and parcel of my life, and no longer represents a constraint. In the same fashion, I have progressively come to consider sport as physical exercise, as a way of being rather than a series of training events.

MEDITATION AND PERFORMANCE

As an athlete, performance is so important that it can also be undermining. Setting objectives exposes us to disappointment and defeat. Philosophy helps me to get out of high-level sport all that is positive, in particular, motivation and focus, without being vulnerable to the rest. Mindfulness plays an essential role during a competition. You are totally absorbed by it, and the impact of doubt and negative thoughts increases progressively. This is all the more the case with a decathlon, because you have to sustain high performance levels despite extreme fatigue. Your mental state is therefore often decisive. You need to stay focused even when you are exhausted. That is what's really at stake. You have to perform a beautiful jump or a beautiful shot while managing the positive and negative thoughts that overwhelm you at that moment. Athletics often allows you three attempts, the third one being your last chance to accomplish a feat. It is then crucial that you succeed in brushing off doubt and pushing back all external pressure that you may feel. Another technique I use is to completely rationalise a situation.

I don't often come across hard-core Buddhists in my sporting discipline. I sometimes meet devout American believers who have trouble reconciling their Christian values with the extreme competitiveness of high-level sport. Indeed, some give up their career in athletics for that reason. Each top-tier athlete has to rely on his concentration, his capacity to focus and his mental training, and mindfulness sessions and yoga have indeed progressively made their way into training programmes. I don't formally do yoga, but my warm-up training includes a few brief wellbeing exercises that I carry out in a meditative state. This is how I am watchful of the signals my body sends me. Since 2016, I have let my body and mind recover in between each event with a 10-minute routine that I designed myself. Most of the time, I lie on my back and I do a few breathing exercises as well as a body scan from top to toe. My muscles then fully relax and I can prepare for the following discipline.

OTHER MINDFULNESS TECHNIQUES

Visualisation is often used by top athletes. Personally, I use my own rather quirky technique. I don't visualise images, but sensations: I feel the movements. In the morning I sometimes do breathing exercises with the help of the PranaBreath app. This app indicates when to breathe with subtle sounds, so that you can find your own rhythm of breathing. I also try to lower my heartbeat using a heartbeat monitor and I usually succeed. Last year I tried out the so-called 'inner fire' meditation for a while. It is a technique that consists of visualising a beam of energy that runs through your spine. I also keep a diary. In a little notebook I jot down my resolutions, my ideas, or a mantra that I want to abide by for a full week or a month. I try, for instance, to be less on the defensive or more open to other people's ideas. I write it down in my notebook so that I can reread it every morning and evening.

PERSONAL RECOMMENDATION

The most important message I would like to pass on is the following: don't make your life complicated! Your initial emotion is triggered by an event and the following emotions by your interpretation of this event. If a situation seems difficult, don't make it even more so. Do this for yourself and for others. That's a good place to start.

TESTIMONIAL: WOUTER TORFS

'The mind is in a constant state of flux and if you
take each thought at face value that's a sure recipe
to become unhappy very rapidly.'

~

*Wouter Torfs is the director of a large Belgian shoe company and in 2019 he
was awarded the Best Employer in Europe prize by the Great Place to Work
Institute. How did he achieve this? His almost tangible charisma and his
candid kindness, which he displayed when we worked together on this book,
gave me some clues, but I also discovered that meditation has helped him in
his various capacities, as a man, a father, a spouse, successful entrepreneur
and award-winning CEO.*

MEDITATION AND PERSONAL DEVELOPMENT

Personal development has been very important to me for quite a few years
now. I enjoy trying out new techniques, but meditation is a continuous presence in my life. I started doing it when I was 35 and was inspired to take up
the practice by my mother. The great classics of meditation literature were
piled up on our living room table. When I was a child during the swinging
60s my mother was already doing Zen meditation. At times she would go
on a weekend retreat at a local monastery, but she would also go to India
for a couple of weeks. She is now 85 and still meditates. She is the one who
passed on to me the need for an eternal quest.

As an adolescent, I could not have cared less about meditation. But as the
years went by, I felt less and less happy, when really I had no reason to
be unhappy. This is how my quest for personal development started. My
coach suggested that I read a book on meditation, as these were the days
before Google. Today there are an overwhelming number of books and texts
on mindfulness available, but in the late eighties, mindfulness was more of
a curiosity. My own practice is more akin to the Zen tradition, where the
emphasis is on posture, the lotus position in particular, which requires you
to hold your back straight.

I focused on my breathing and I observed my thoughts whirling around. I thus became aware that my 'monkey mind' was hopping from one topic to another and breaking up my train of thought. The mind is in a constant state of flux and if you take each thought at face value that's a sure recipe to becoming unhappy very rapidly. I would meditate in the morning for 20 minutes, which became a habit I still sustain. Not every day, but for sure when I don't feel too good about myself or when I know that I have a hard day ahead of me. I don't use a timer. Instead, when I feel I have done enough, I try to continue for a little longer. In general, I tend to sleep really well. And when I don't, it is often due to stress. I then need to sit on my little mat and look that stress straight in the eye.

MINDFULNESS AND FAMILY

Over the years, my wife came round to the idea of trying it out and now we sometimes meditate together. She loves Headspace. As teenagers, my kids rejected the whole personal development idea. It seemed totally absurd to them. When I was a teenager, the spiritual world of my mother didn't attract me. Yet, nowadays my daughters have developed an interest. One of them is really passionate about mindfulness and has completed a training programme in it.

BUDDHISTS AND CHRISTIANS

I would not say that I have become a Buddhist, but I am certainly attracted to Buddhist thought. I have attended a few retreats. The fact that you are invited to live with monks and join in their rhythm is very soothing. For me, Buddhism is not a religion, but more a method that allows me to grow and that offers ethical values akin to Christian ones, like 'Thou shalt not kill', 'Thou shalt not lie'. I do like to take part in Buddhist rituals, but I don't per se feel the need for it. As a Catholic, I observe Christian values, but I recognise in Buddhism many elements that have been progressively erased from Catholicism, because they represent rituals that are too formal.

NON-DUALITY

Meditation is a catch-all concept that encompasses different types of practice and philosophical traditions. You need to find your own way among those. With all due respect to them, visualisation and mantras have not done much for me. I started with Zen meditation mindfulness and then turned towards mindfulness, whereas now I am exploring the idea of non-duality with a professor in Tibetan Buddhism. He teaches introspective meditation, which is different from soothing meditation. In introspective meditation, the aim is to try and become aware that your mind is endowed with content, thoughts and emotions in particular, but that the essence of your being is consciousness. It is an awareness of awareness. It allows you to progressively develop a new relationship with reality. Meditation helps us to relax, but also not to mistake our emotions and thoughts for reality. We are not the sum of our emotions, but the result of our consciousness.

WORK, LEADERSHIP AND MEDITATION

Meditation has allowed me to smooth things out as man and as an entrepreneur. When you accept the idea that everything is interwoven, including us humans, it is easier to accept others and the advice they give. That is a crucial and invaluable characteristic in a boss. The quality of presence, the degree to which one is in the here and now of the present, also plays a key role in a professional setting, in particular when it comes to presentations and meetings. I often see business leaders who are distracted and let their thoughts stray. They lose the connection with the present moment. How can thoughts, sensations and feelings be real? Meditation also allows you to have a better grasp of moments of tension and conflict. However painful or excessive the emotions feel, they are only transitory. Once you understand that, you are in a better position to manage situations you encounter rather than simply enduring them. Meditation also allows you to build resilience in a very competitive system. It allows you to keep your feet on the ground. I am prone to overthinking and loosing myself in my thoughts. Meditation is the perfect foil to that.

MEDITATING CEOS

Twice a year, we organise a two-day CEO conference with six other business leaders who have now become good friends. These meeting have grown into platforms where we share and exchange ideas on all possible fundamental questions, whether personal or professional. The programme, which always schedules in a half-hour of silence, originated with the idea of a 'sacred place' where people could meet and meet fully. Meditation has not really become a new fashion among CEOs, I believe, but I admit it is a growing movement.

Access to mindfulness and giving it one's own meaning has become much more widespread

MINDFULNESS FOR EMPLOYEES
In my business we offer open training. This means that staff can take up three training programmes a year paid for by the company, in a domain that may be totally unrelated to their professional activity. It may be healthy cooking, photography or mindfulness. The idea behind this scheme is that developing personal talents makes people happier.

ENTREPRENEURSHIP, ORIENTAL PHILOSOPHY AND BURNOUT
Love is the DNA of our business. It is what binds us to each other and what binds us to our clients. We prefer to nourish it rather than to capitalise it. We do not consider our employees to be people whose services we are renting for the skills they bring in. We welcome people as a whole, with their dreams, their talents, their deficiencies, their expectations and their anxieties. I watch over my staff with a benevolent gaze that stems from the Oriental contemplative traditions. When people suffer from burnout, it is the thinking system that takes control and therefore hampers their development.

People seem to believe that they can cope by thinking more or better. During convalescence, meditation can be of great help, but when the crisis hits, I doubt that is the case. However, I do know co-workers who, with the help of a mindfulness therapist, have been able to get back on track.

SILENCE FOR PEACE
Last but not least: silence is golden. After the Brussels and Paris terrorist attacks, the debate solidified around an 'us versus them' dichotomy. Voices from the left and right of the political spectrum expressed themselves, but silence was the big absentee in the debate. That's why we had the initiative Silence for Peace. We organised a sit-in in Brussels where we invited the whole population, regardless of their political or religious persuasions, to come and join us and sit in silence. We repeat this initiative each year in a different major city.

~

THE RESOURCE PROJECT

From 2013 to 2016, my colleague, Professor Tania Singer, from the Social Neuroscience Lab in Berlin, carried out the ReSource Project. With more than 300 participants, it is one of the largest scientific studies on the mental trainability of qualities such as mindfulness, compassion, perspective-taking and pro-social behaviours. The principal goal of Tania's programme is the scientific evaluation of the effects of different types of mental practices on our psychological and physical health. The nine-month longitudinal mental training study compared exercises focusing on: (1) present-moment attention and sensing the internal state of your body; (2) compassion and loving-kindness training; and (3) learning to control your mental processes and perspective-taking of yourself and others.

At present, more than 40 scientific papers have been published based on the studied cohort in the ReSource Project. They observed evidence for differential training effects of the mental exercises; measurements ranged from structural brain changes measured by MRI to improvements in social intelligence, altruism and stress-hormone responses. Tania and her team from the German Max Planck Society demonstrated that you can, even as an adult, change and improve your mental wellbeing and social intelligence — but it matters what type of meditation you practise.

All tested practices reduced stress, enhanced attention and improved altruism and cooperation, but affective training was the best way to increase compassion. Social stress levels decreased by over 50 per cent and meditating with a partner was especially effective in reducing cortisol stress levels. The meditation exercises visibly increased the volume of grey matter in brain networks related to attention and emotional control. Participants felt happier and more energised; more present in the moment; more aware of their body; more aware of their thoughts and the 'little voice' in their head; more able to disengage from distracting thoughts; were more positive about other people; felt more socially close and connected and more empathetic and compassionate towards themselves and towards others. Compassion-meditation increased objectively measured levels of altruistic behaviours like charitable donation, trust and generosity.

Chapter 11

Tools and tips

~

'When more than 30 years ago, a few pioneering
Western medics tried to introduce meditation in the
traditional health system, the people they worked
with mocked them. But this did not put them off. They
choose instead to call it 'mindfulness' rather than
'meditation' and got on with their research.'

— ANDY PUDDICOMBE, Founder of Headspace

If, having read this book, you decide to dedicate more time to the present moment and the nature of your thoughts, then that's great news! And technology is there to help you. There are a number of meditation apps out there that are very popular, some of which I have already mentioned. There are also different exercises that offer real-time biofeedback. This biological feedback, where detectors measure your brain activity, informs you of the results and therefore helps you learn to control the activity in question![1]

One is perfectly entitled to be critical about the commercial exploitation of meditation. Just as one is rightly entitled to question the use of technology within a practice that seeks to avoid all forms of distraction. That being said, I remain convinced of the usefulness of such tools, in particular because in my own case I found them helpful and because I hear from many of the patients I see in my outpatient clinic that they have experienced the added value of these tools. Meditation apps can be used as a springboard to set up your own mental training programme, in the same way as sports programmes such as Start2Run, Nike Plus, Runkeeper, Formyfit, Fitbit and many others have encouraged people to take up jogging or make sure they do their 10,000 steps a day. Personally, I find this a very positive development. Recent controlled trials that employed a mindfulness meditation app also demonstrated measurable reductions in stress, anxiety, depression and psychological wellbeing.[2]

Click and meditate

Like many others, I tried out different guided meditation exercises on my smartphone and I still do that today. Apps allow people to check their statistics, their progress, and remind them of the objectives they have set for themselves. These apps are often free to start with, but after a while you have to pay in order to continue using them or you need to purchase a subscription.

You can now choose between a dazzling 2,500 mobile applications for guidance in taking care of your mental health and tranquillity. I would propose you try some out for yourselves and choose which type of voice, accent and language makes you feel most comfortable and at what price.

The first app I would like to discuss is called Imagine Clarity. It is a very successful English-speaking app created by my friend Matthieu Ricard and Dr Alan Wallace. It focuses mainly on loving kindness meditation and encourages users to develop a more meaningful life. The app offers videos with exercise sessions and inspirational classes led by Matthieu. In his own words, 'Imagine Clarity has been designed with and framed by a secular ethics, with the purpose of helping you to become a better human being capable of more kindness.'

For beginners, a nice app is Petit BamBou, which offers free access to a basic class, as well as to great videos that take you through the basic concepts of mindfulness. If you want to continue, you will have to purchase the paid-for version. The modules allow you explore different topics, such as stress and anxiety. Petit BamBou is the leading European mindfulness app with 7 million users and offers guided exercises in English, French, Dutch, German, Spanish and Italian.

Another European companion on the journey to inner peace is the Mindfulness App. It offers programs for anyone who wants to sleep better, worry less, and have stronger relationships. With more than 250 meditations and courses from some of the world's most renowned meditation teachers, there is something for everyone. Whether you're a sceptical beginner or a more experienced meditation practitioner, it takes you on a journey towards a calmer, more peaceful life.

The most popular app worldwide is Headspace. It was launched in 2010 and has achieved 46 million users around the world. By 2020, the app could be seen as a series on Netflix, had over 2 million paid subscribers and more than 600 businesses were using its on-the-job mental wellness tool. The voice that guides you through the meditation sessions is that of Andy Puddicombe, one of the founders of Headspace, who gave up his career as a sports coach in order to put on the robe of a Buddhist monk. Recently I had the opportunity to use a version of Headspace adapted for the small screen of a Canadian Airlines flight. In my opinion, this version is ideally tailored to people who suffer from fear of flying. As of 2021, it offers the possibility to choose between English, French, German, Spanish and Portuguese.

Calm is an app that deserves to be better known. It offers many of the same perks as Headspace, such as options to download meditations for offline streaming. Calm also offers Apple Health integration, tracking the number of minutes each day you spend meditating, if you're into that, which is a

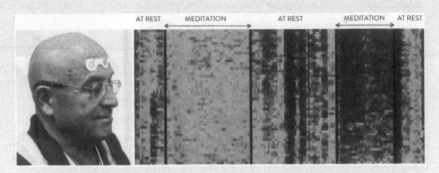

AT REST　　MEDITATION　　AT REST　　MEDITATION　AT REST

© Steven Laureys, with warm thanks to our colleague, professor in mathematics,
Nathan Intrator (Tel-Aviv University/Neurosteer).

'Our mind behaves like a captive monkey who, in his agitation, becomes more and more entangled in his bonds.'
MATTHIEU RICARD

New technologies now allow us to track live the fluctuations of electrical waves or EEG in the brain with just a simple band that is stuck on the forehead.

We can here see in black and white – in reality it would be all the colours of the rainbow – how, when he is 'at rest', constantly mutating thoughts and emotions run through Matthieu Ricard's brain. We all experience this phenomenon, but it is more controlled in trained monks. At times these thoughts concerning the future or the past can be disturbing and can linger. This is what is called rehashing. Our brain can't help it: it thinks continually. Even when we sleep our brain cells are still very active (as we have studied in our research lab). These mental experiences are in constant flux, just like the waves of the ocean. In the picture you can see how the black waves come and go.

During this effortless presence meditation session, we can see how the brain activity is characterised by a certain stability. The colours are light and solid, and there are fewer 'chaotic' EEG waves, just like a very calm sea, with fewer of the jumps created by sudden, brisk thoughts. However, there are different meditation techniques, just as there are different sports, each of which has their own specific brain characteristics. For instance, during the second meditation period illustrated here, Matthieu is practising loving kindness meditation. This translates into darker colours that are again more stable than the whirlwind induced by the normal state of wakefulness, when our conscious experiences seem to be all over the place.

Some of these very simple measuring devices are already available on the market, like for instance the Muse band (see page 198). This gives beginners data about what happens in their brain during meditation and therefore allows them to improve more rapidly. Most of us don't need this, though. Taking a few minutes entirely dedicated to yourself by sitting comfortably in a chair or on a cushion and doing your favourite meditation exercises is entirely sufficient as far as I am concerned. Meditating informally on the bus, tram or at work is perfectly fine too.[3]

common feature for many apps now. It offers guided sessions of meditation, soothing music and stories to help you fall asleep. As of 2021, Calm was available in English, German, French, Spanish, Korean, Portuguese and Japanese.

In the pragmatic category, the app Ten Percent Happier has a special place. It is linked to the podcast of the same name, hosted by Dan Harris, which offers fascinating interviews with guests such as the Dalai Lama, Matthieu Ricard, Jon Kabat–Zinn and Daniel Goleman. This app has the advantage over others in that it offers personalised coaching alongside learning videos and guided meditation sessions. What's more, you can ask your own questions at any time and have a conversation with a mindfulness coach who has at least ten years of experience under their belt. This is theoretically available within a day (I did not try this feature myself).

Waking Up is another interesting app, created by the neuroscientist, philosopher and seasoned meditator Sam Harris who invited me onto his popular podcast (of which more on page 39). Known for his unshakable faith in the potential of science, he has published several books that advocate a form of spirituality stripped of all religious dimensions. For him meditation is not simply about fighting stress: it can fundamentally contribute to changing our view of the world. In his app, you will need to go through 50 introductory modules before getting access to the daily meditation sessions.

I have also tried out Insight Timer, which is a sort of social media platform for those who do meditation. Besides offering a map of who is meditating at the same time as you, you can also see who is meditating nearby and invite friends to join and meditate together. The personalised timer is interesting for those who are more experienced and it offers the nice pleasant sound of a singing bowl. You can also plan short meditation sessions when you are travelling, set background noises, and it also offers a choice of several coaches.

Finally, I also use the breathe function on my Apple Watch, which, I grant you, is an expensive device. This function allows you to know when it is time to work on your breathing and to breathe mindfully seven times in a row. I also use it in the morning before I get up. The vibrations on my wrist guide me through my deep breathing over a period of one to five minutes and allow me to see how my heart rate immediately slows down. Android and GooglePlay offer similar systems. A more recent and very pleasant personal discovery is the (Belgian) Moonbird. Life device – it looks like a small avocado – that you take in your hand and which measures your heart rate. Based on that, it calculates the right rhythm for you to breathe in and out. The device will then expand and contract at that rate, so that you automatically take over the rhythm. A cool and very intuitive way to guide your meditation breathing exercises and give you direct feedback.

Muse

Muse is not an app, but a portable device like an Apple Watch, Fitbit bracelet or a pedometer. This band captures brain activity and sends the data to an app that you can download to your smartphone. It is an interesting technological tool that shows in real time what happens in your brain. When you meditate you may, for instance, hear sounds that occur outdoors in nature. The quieter you are, the more soothing this is. In this way, you are immediately warned when your thoughts are straying. It is a nice example of the gamification of meditation.

In our lab at Liège, we use Neurosteer, which was designed by my friend and colleague Professor Nathan Intrator, a mathematician at the University of Tel-Aviv, who also designed a piece of technology similar to Muse that you just stick on your forehead. The system measures the electrical activity of the brain and translates the data into various states, such as restlessness or watchfulness. These states can be visualised with different colour codes, so the constantly evolving patches of colour reveal to what extent the mind is wandering. Of course, we couldn't resist the temptation to test this device on Matthieu Ricard's forehead. The results were mind-boggling. If you compare Matthieu to the ordinary mortal, the difference is overwhelming. We also tested him during several conferences I gave with Matthieu, at the Philharmonic Hall in Liège and the Centre of Fine Arts in Brussels. The public could see how Matthieu was able to modify the electrical activity in his brain at a moment's notice. And we could all watch that being translated on the screen, with the colours remaining uniformly stable. It was incredible! We got similar results with other experts like Lama Zeupa at the Yeunten Ling Tibetan Institute in Huy.

~

Chapter 12

In defence of wonder

~

'I beg you to have patience with everything
unresolved in your heart and to try to love the
questions themselves as if they were locked rooms
or books written in a very foreign language'

– RAINER MARIA RILKE, writer, poet and Austrian mystic, 1875–1926

Nobody in life is spared difficult moments. If happiness were with us on a permanent basis, we would not know what it meant. Joy and wellbeing are measured against moments that are less pleasant. There will always be moments when you are less comfortable and when you might need to fight to survive. For me, that was the moment when I suddenly found myself alone, emotionally shattered and in charge of three kids, while juggling the demands of a full-time job. But the good news is that there are techniques and skills that can help you keep your head above water. As far as I am concerned, I discovered long-distance running, yoga, meditation and Matthieu Ricard, and I was capable of loving again.

Over 20 years ago, one of my psychiatrist colleagues told me, 'It is not reality that matters, it is the way you experience reality.' This little sentence helped me understand many things. And this type of realisation can literally transform your life. When you meditate and are fully aware of things, you analyse the nature of the events you are going through. You do so by observing your thoughts, perceptions and emotions, so that you can take stock and manage them better. Matthieu advises you remain alert and react rapidly. He compares emotions with a spark that can turn into a huge blaze and set a whole forest on fire. The more you are able to observe these sparks, the earlier you recognise their existence, the better you will be able to let go, take distance, and control them and not let yourself become their blind slave.

It is not reality that matters, it is the way you experience reality.

I hope you are now in a better position to understand the whole potential of meditation. If that isn't the case, be aware that I am not a priest of any sort. I'm not forcing you to meditate every day. But it would be fantastic if you tried out a few formal or informal mindfulness exercises as you read through this book or once you have finished it. Be open-minded and choose something that suits you! When you eat at a sushi bar is it not the same? You choose what you like and leave what you don't. The choice is yours, but let common sense be always with you!

As a scientist, I believe in having a critical mind and I distrust any person, guru or group that claims they hold the only truth. This is all the more the case when it comes to the topic of this book: mindfulness and meditation.

When I read that a certain method is the only authentic one, I go into alarm mode. It is as if a sports teacher tells you that he is the only one able to teach you the rules of the game and that what all the other teachers are teaching is false. Obviously that would be ridiculous! I didn't learn about neurology from one single professor or with one single book. Like everyone else, I obtain my knowledge from a multiplicity of sources. So you can learn meditation in many ways and see what suits you best. Looking at different perspectives and approaches will enrich your learning experience. It will also shield you from any form of dogmatism; any claim to an 'absolute' or 'unshakable' truth. Science evolves continuously and the sources mentioned in this book will inevitably be either confirmed or corrected in the light of new studies or research.

Above all, I invite you to experience meditation for yourself. Reading about the topic, the scientific findings and the testimonies of others (such as those offered in this book) can inspire you and give you knowledge and insights, but you will need to feel the power of meditation for yourself. No one can do it for you. The only true talent you need is the willingness and curiosity to try it out.

Personally, I believe that we underestimate the ways in which science and technology can help progress. To guarantee such progress, it is crucial that we keep up a critical stance, as well as a curious and open mind, but this strictly scientific mindset should not overshadow our sense of spirituality. I marvel at the idea that we are able to contemplate the world in an open-minded and inquisitive spirit. The fact we are all here on earth as unique human beings, yet all linked to one another in this vast universe is something that continuously fascinates me – and despite all our scientific progress we still know so little about this incredible life. It leaves me with a sense of wonder, awe and gratitude.

When it comes to meditation, mindfulness, hypnosis, yoga, Tai Chi, qigong, Autogenic training and sophrology, many of my scientific colleagues are quick to throw the baby out with the bathwater. Admittedly, it is a domain that may resort to pseudo-scientific practices, but sometimes medics don't grant enough value to soft 'complementary' medicine. We learn how to understand and explain specific pathologies, so that we can rapidly classify them into small boxes and prescribe some medication that fits each of those well-defined entities. In my traditional medical training, I was taught very little about non-pharmacological approaches and a more holistic, integrative and preventive medicine. With our health 2.0 system, which is based on cold classifications, strictly defined specialisms, high-tech machines, artificial intelligence computers and robots, we are at risk of losing a global, and human, approach. That is why the so-called alternative medicines have become so popular. In my view, there is only one medicine – the one that helps!

As scientists, sometimes we tend to arrogantly believe that we know (almost) everything. But in all honesty, despite the fantastic progress we have made, the extent of our ignorance of the how and why of the universe, of life and of consciousness is enormous. I force myself to continue to learn, to see the world through the amazed eyes of a curious and open-minded child. When my little Louis takes his shower, he looks with wonder at how water runs down his body. He does not anticipate, as I do, the meeting that will follow. As adults we need to learn to rediscover this sense of wonder, to observe the present moment in the light of it, whether it be the gaze of a dog, the smile of a stranger, the sun that shines, the rain that falls from the sky, the grass that is green or a child that comes into the world...

~

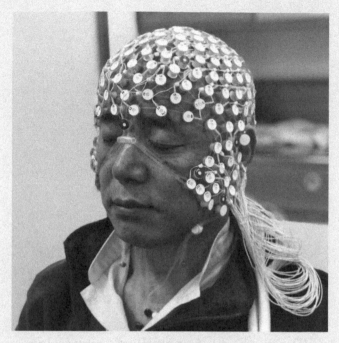

© Steven Laureys

'Whoever dares to let go naturally becomes a person full of gentleness and friendliness, and teaches others to behave with the same warmness.'

LAMA ZEUPA

My dear friend Lama Zeupa is a monk based at the Yeunten Ling Tibetan Institute in Huy, Belgium. Here he is seen in the middle of a mindfulness meditation session, in 'focused attention' meditation to be specific, while our team measures his brain activity.

Meditation, mindfulness and kindred techniques can offer us tools to improve our mental wellbeing and our health in general. As you will have understood, everyone can benefit as long as they approach it with an open, undogmatic mind. There is no need to be or become a mystic or monk. There is no need either to enlist in any cult or sect or find an expensive guru. You can simply take a workshop or classes with a qualified professional or download an app on your smartphone, read a book with an audio guide or watch a video on the Internet to start your own mental health programme – an 'I am meditating for good shape' programme of sorts. Formal meditation, which means you are sitting on a cushion in the lotus position, is just one way of doing things. But you may also do it informally, whenever you have a 'lost' moment during your day. How it precisely works in the brain is only partially known, but many studies have evidenced the numerous direct or indirect benefits: fewer negative thoughts, less rehashing, less stress, better sleep, better immunity, lower blood pressure, decreased pain and fewer depressive relapses... The list is long and there are few risks or negative side-effects. So why not give it a try?

'Wisdom is about understanding that
all you see, all you feel, is as ephemeral
as a dream, an illusion or light
in the night.
The method is to be full of compassion
for all beings; in a nutshell, it is to have
a good heart.
Without wisdom, you misperceive
everything and without compassion,
your wisdom is not worth much.'

— MATTHIEU RICARD

Notes

~

Foreword

1. Chételat G. et al., 2017, 'Reduced age-associated brain changes in expert meditators: A multimodal neuroimaging pilot study', *Scientific Reports*, 7(1), p. 10160 ; Marchant N.L. et al., 2018, 'Effects of a mindfulness-based intervention versus health education on mental health in patients with subjective cognitive decline', *Alzheimers Dement* (NY), 14(4), pp. 737–745; André C. et al. Medit-Ageing Research Group, 2020, 'Association of Sleep-Disordered Breathing With Alzheimer Disease Biomarkers in Community-Dwelling Older Adults', *JAMA Neurol.* 77(6), pp. 716–724.

2. Rinpoche Y. M. and Swanson E., 2009, *The Joy of Living: Unlocking the Secret and Science of Happiness*, New York: Harmony Books.

3. Ricard M. and Singer W., 2017, *Beyond the Self: Conversations Between Buddhism and Neuroscience*, Cambridge: MIT Press.

Introduction

1. Bodart O., Fecchio M., Massimini M., Wannez S., Virgillito A., Casarotto S., Rosanova M., Lutz A., Ricard M., Laureys S. and Gosseries O., 2018, 'Meditation-induced modulation of brain response to transcranial magnetic stimulation', *Brain Stimulation*, 11(6), pp. 1397–1400.

Chapter 1 Happiness within reach... of your brain!

1. Goyal M., Singh S., Sibinga E.M. et al., 2014, 'Meditation programs for psychological stress and wellbeing: A systematic review and meta–analysis', *JAMA Internal Medicine*, 174(3), pp. 357–368.

2. Vella E. and McIver S., 2019, 'Reducing stress and burnout in the public-sector work environment: A mindfulness meditation pilot study', *Health Promotion Journal of Australia*, 30(2), pp. 219–227.

3. Zhou E. S., Gardiner P., and Bertisch S. M., 2017, 'Integrative medicine for insomnia', *Medical Clinics of North America*, 101(5), pp. 865–879.

4. Nahin R. L., Boineau R., Khalsa P. S., Stussman B. J. and Weber W. J., 2016, 'Evidence-based evaluation of complementary health approaches for pain management in the United States', *Mayo Clinic Proceedings*, 91(9), pp. 1292–1306.

5. Brook R. D., Jackson E. A., Giorgini P., and McGowan C. L., 2015, 'When and how to recommend "alternative approaches" in the management of high blood pressure', *American Journal of Medicine*, 128(6), pp. 567–570.

6. Heckenberg R. A., Eddy P., Kent S. and Wright B. J., 2018, 'Do workplace-based mindfulness meditation programs improve physiological indices of stress? A systematic review and meta-analysis', *Journal of Psychosomatic Research*, 114, pp. 62–71.

Chapter 3 A close-up of your brilliant brain

1. Fox K. C. et al., 2014, 'Is meditation associated with altered brain structure? A systematic review and meta-analysis of morphometric neuroimaging in meditation practitioners', *Neuroscience and Biobehavioral Reviews*, 43, pp. 48–73; Fox K. C. et al., 2016, 'Functional neuroanatomy of meditation: A review and meta-analysis of 78 functional neuroimaging investigations', *Neuroscience and Biobehavioral Reviews*, 65, pp. 208–228.

2. Sharma K. et al., 2018, 'Enhanced white matter integrity in corpus callosum of long-term Brahmakumaris Rajayoga meditators', *Brain Connectivity*, 2018, 8(1), pp. 49–55.

3. Levenson R. W., Ekman P. and Ricard M., 2012, 'Meditation and the startle response: A case study', *Emotion*, 12(3), pp. 650–658.

4. Tang Y. Y., Hölzel B. K. and Posner M. I., 2015, 'The neuroscience of mindfulness meditation', *Nature Reviews Neuroscience*, 16(4), pp. 213–225.

5. One should not limit the complex processes that are activated by attention and emotions to one area of the brain. Similarly, it would be equally restrictive to attribute functions, such as language or creativity, to just one area of the brain. We are constantly using all areas of the brain.

6. Chételat G. et al., 2017, 'Reduced age-associated brain changes in expert meditators: A multimodal neuroimaging pilot study', *Scientific Reports*, 7(1).

7. Lutz A., Greischar L. L., Rawlings N. B., Ricard M. and Davidson R. J., 2004, 'Long-term meditators self-induce high-amplitude gamma synchrony during mental practice', *Proceedings of the National Academy of Sciences of the United States of America*, 16, 101(46), pp. 16369–16373.

8. Bodart O., Fecchio M., Massimini M., Wannez S., Virgillito A., Casarotto S., Rosanova M., Lutz A., Ricard M., Laureys S. and Gosseries O., 2018, 'Meditation-induced modulation of brain response to transcranial magnetic stimulation', *Brain Stimulation*, 11(6), pp. 1397–1400.

9. Ibid.

10. Davidson R. J. and McEwen B. S., 2012, 'Social influences on neuroplasticity: Stress and interventions to promote well-being', *Nature Neuroscience*, 15(5), pp. 689–695.

11. Hölzel B. K. et al., 2010, 'Stress reduction correlates with structural changes in the amygdala', *Social, Cognitive and Affective Neuroscience*, 5, pp. 11–17.

12. Singer T. and Engert V., 2018, 'It matters what you practice: Differential training effects on subjective experience, behavior, brain and body in the ReSource Project', *Current Opinion in Psychology*, 28, pp. 151–158.

13. Hasenkamp W. and Barsalou L. W., 2012, 'Effects of meditation experience on functional connectivity of distributed brain networks', *Frontiers in Human Neuroscience*, 6, article ID 38.

14. Ricard M., Lutz A. and Davidson R. J., 2014, 'Mind of the meditator', *Scientific American*, 311(5), pp. 38–45.

15. Brefczynski-Lewis J. A., Lutz A., Schaefer H. S., Levinson D. B. and Davidson R. J., 2007, 'Neural correlates of attentional expertise in long-term meditation practitioners', *Proceedings of the National Academy of Sciences of the United States of America*, 104(27), pp. 11483–11488.

16. Killingsworth M. A. and Gilbert D. T., 2010, 'A wandering mind is an unhappy mind', *Science*, 330(6006), p. 932.

17. Hanh, T. N., 2015, *How to Walk*, Berkeley: Parallax Press.

Chapter 4 To all those who are impatient and highly sceptical

1. Kreplin U., Farias M. and Brazil I. A., 2018, 'The limited prosocial effects of meditation: A systematic review and meta-analysis', *Scientific Reports*, 8(1), p. 2403.

2. Gotink R. A. et al., 2016, '8-week mindfulness-based stress reduction induces brain changes similar to traditional long-term meditation practice: A systematic review', *Brain and Cognition*, 108, pp. 32–41.

3. Van Dam N. T. et al., 2018, 'Mind the hype: A critical evaluation and prescriptive agenda for research on mindfulness and meditation', *Perspectives on Psychological Science*, 13(1), pp. 36–61.

4. Thompson E. and Varela F. J., 2001, 'Radical embodiment: neural dynamics and consciousness', *Trends in Cognitive Sciences*, 5(10), pp. 418–425.

5. Dahl C. J. and Davidson R. J., 2018, 'Mindfulness and the contemplative life: Pathways to connection, insight and purpose', *Current Opinion in Psychology*, 28, pp. 60–64.

6. King B. G., Conklin Q. A., Zanesco A. P. and Saron C. D., 2019, 'Residential meditation retreats: Their role in contemplative practice and significance for psychological research', *Current Opinions in Psychology*, 28, pp. 238–244.

7. Paulson S., Davidson R., Jha A. and Kabat-Zinn J., 2013, 'Becoming conscious: The science of mindfulness', *Annals of the New York Academy of Sciences*, 1303, pp. 87–104.

8. Singer T. and Engert V., 2019, 'It matters what you practice: Differential training effects on subjective experience, behavior, brain and body in the ReSource Project', *Current Opinions in Psychology*, 28, pp. 151–158.

9. Turan B. et al., 2015, 'Anticipatory sensitization to repeated stressors: The role of initial cortisol reactivity and meditation/emotion skills training', *Psychoneuroendocrinology*, 52, pp. 229–238.

10. Jha A. P. et al., 2019, 'Does mindfulness training help working memory "work" better?', *Current Opinions in Psychology*, 28, pp. 273–278.

11. Lutz A. et al., 2018, 'The Age-Well observational study on expert meditators in the Medit-Ageing European project', *Alzheimers and Dementia*, 4, pp. 756–764.

12. This work is being carried out in collaboration with formidable colleagues, such as Bindu Kutty, Professor in Neurophysiology at the National Institute of Mental Health and Neurosciences (NIMHANS) in Bangalore, India; engineer Rajanikant Panda (Panda R. et al., 2016, 'Temporal dynamics of the default mode network characterize meditation–induced alterations in consciousness', *Frontiers in Human Neuroscience*, 10, p. 372), who is currently finishing his doctoral thesis in our team; anaesthetist Subramaniam Balachundhar at Harvard University, who works on the effects of yoga on the brain; my friend the psychologist Ron Kupers at the University of Copenhagen and his spouse Dr Laurence Dricot from the Catholic University of Leuven, who studies the effects of heartfulness meditation compared to physical exercise; and, of course, Matthieu himself and the scientists

of Mind & Life Europe, in particular Antoine Lutz, a mindfulness pioneer at the University of Lyon.

13. This has been evidenced by a whole series of research studies carried out around the world, but mostly in the United-States, as is shown in the chart on page 81.

14. Bodart O. et al., 2018, 'Meditation-induced modulation of brain response to transcranial magnetic stimulation', *Brain Stimulation*, 11 (6), pp. 1397–1400.

15. Gosseries O. et al., 2015, 'On the cerebral origin of EEG responses to TMS: Insights from severe cortical lesions', *Brain Stimulation*, 8 (1), pp. 142–149.

16. Comolatti R et al., 2019, 'A fast and general method to empirically estimate the complexity of brain responses to transcranial and intracranial stimulations', *Brain Stimulation*, 12(5), pp. 1280–1289.

Chapter 5 The benefits of meditation on body and mind

1. Levine G. N. et al., 2017, 'Meditation and cardiovascular risk reduction: A scientific statement from the American Heart Association', *Journal of the American Heart Association*, 6 (10), pii: e002218.

2. Mindfulness cognitive-based therapy (MCBT) is a psychotherapy approach which combines cognitive behaviour therapy (CBT) with mindfulness meditation exercises.

3. The number of studies quoted in the database of clinical studies financed by both the public and private sectors around the world since 1999.

4. Tang Y. Y., Hölzel B. K. and Posner M. I., 2015, 'The neuroscience of mindfulness meditation', *Nature Reviews Neuroscience*, 16(4), pp. 213–225.

5. Gaylord S. A., et al., 2011, 'Mindfulness training reduces the severity of irritable bowel syndrome in women: Results of a randomized controlled trial', *American Journal of Gastroenterology*, 106(9), pp. 1678–1688.

6. US National Institute on Drug Abuse 2018.

7. Belgian Pharmaceutical Association, 2016.

8. French National Agency for the Safety of Medication, 2018.

9. Veehof M. M., Oskam M. J., Schreurs K. M. G. and Bohlmeijer E. T., 2011, 'Acceptance-based interventions for the treatment of chronic pain. A systematic review and meta–analysis', *Pain*, 152, pp. 533–542.

10. Zhang M. F., Wen Y. S., Liu W. Y., Peng L. F., Wu X. D. and Liu Q. W., 2015, 'Effectiveness of mindfulness-based therapy for reducing anxiety and depression in patients with cancer: A meta-analysis', *Medicine (Baltimore)*, 94(45), e0897–0.

11. Black D. S., Peng C., Sleight A. G., Nguyen N., Lenz H. J. and Figueiredo J. C., 2017, 'Mindfulness practice reduces cortisol blunting during chemotherapy: A randomized controlled study of colorectal cancer patients', *Cancer*, 123(16), pp. 3088–3096.

12. Day M. A. et al., 2019, 'A pilot randomized controlled trial comparing mindfulness meditation, cognitive therapy and mindfulness-based cognitive therapy for chronic low back pain', *Pain Medicine*, 20(11), pp. 2134–2148.

13. Grant J. A., Courtemanche J., Duerden E. G., Duncan G. H. and Rainville P., 2010, 'Cortical thickness and pain sensitivity in Zen meditators', *Emotion*, 10(1), pp. 43–53.

14. Lutz A., McFarlin D. R., Perlman D. M., Salomons T. V. and Davidson R. J., 2013, 'Altered anterior insula activation during anticipation and experience of painful stimuli in expert meditators', *NeuroImage*, 64, pp. 538–546; Perlman D. M., Salomons T. V., Davidson R. J. and Lutz A., 2010, 'Differential effects on pain intensity and unpleasantness of two meditation practices', *Emotion*, 10(1), p. 65; May L. M., Kosek P., Zeidan F. and Berkman E. T., 2018, 'Enhancement of meditation analgesia by opioid antagonist in experienced meditators', *Psychosomatic Medicine*, 80(9), pp. 807–813.

15. Garland S. N., Zhou E. S., Gonzalez B. D. and Rodriguez N., 2016, 'The quest for mindful sleep: A critical synthesis of the impact of mindfulness-based interventions for insomnia', *Current Sleep Medicine Reports*, 2(3), pp. 142–150.

16. Pagnoni G. and Cekic M., 2007, 'Age effects on gray matter volume and attentional performance in Zen meditation', *Neurobiology of Aging*, 28(10), pp. 1623–1627.

17. Conklin Q. A., Crosswell A. D., Saron C. D. and Epel E. S., 2018, 'Meditation, stress processes and telomere biology', *Current Opinion in Psychology*, 28, pp. 92–101.

18. Chételat G. et al., 2017, 'Reduced age-associated brain changes in expert meditators: A multimodal neuroimaging pilot study', *Scientific Reports*, 7(1), p. 10160.

19. Conklin Q., King B., Zanesco A., Pokorny J., Hamidi A., Lin J., Epel E., Blackburn E. and Saron C., 2015, 'Telomere lengthening after three weeks of an intensive insight meditation retreat', *Psychoneuroendocrinology*, 61, pp. 26–27; Jacobs T. L., Epel E. S., Lin J., Blackburn E. H., Wolkowitz O. M., Bridwell D. A. and Saron C. D., 2011, 'Intensive meditation training, immune cell telomerase activity and psychological mediators', *Psychoneuroendocrinology*, 36(5), pp. 664–681; Sahdra B. K., MacLean K. A., Ferrer E., Shaver P. R., Rosenberg E. L., Jacobs T. L. and Saron C. D., 2011, 'Enhanced response inhibition during intensive meditation training predicts improvements in self-reported adaptive socioemotional functioning', *Emotion*, 11(2), pp. 299–312.

20. Conklin Q. A. et al., 2018, 'Meditation, stress processes, and telomere biology', *Current Opinion in Psychology*, 28, pp. 92–101; Buric et al., 2017, 'What is the molecular signature of mind-body interventions? A systematic review of gene expression changes induced by meditation and related practices', *Frontiers in Immunology*, 8, p. 670.

21. Tang Y. Y., Hölzel B. K. and Posner M. I., 2015, 'The neuroscience of mindfulness meditation', *Nature Reviews Neuroscience*, 16(4), pp. 213–225.

22. Sapolsky R. M., 1998, *Why Zebras Don't Get Ulcers: An Updated Guide To Stress, Stress Related Diseases and Coping*, New York: W. H. Freeman, second edition.

23. Kral T. R. A., Schuyler B. S., Mumford J. A., Rosenkranz M. A., Lutz A. and Davidson R. J., 2018, 'Impact of short- and long-term mindfulness meditation training on amygdala reactivity to emotional stimuli', *NeuroImage*, 181, pp. 301–313.

24. Creswell J. D. et al., 2016, 'Alterations in resting-state functional connectivity link mindfulness meditation with reduced interleukin-6: A randomized controlled trial', *Biological Psychiatry*, 80(1), pp. 53–61.

25. Kaliman P. et al., 2014, 'Rapid changes in histone deacetylases and inflammatory gene expression in expert meditators', *Psychoneuroendocrinology*, 40,

pp. 96–107; Pace T. W. W. et al., 2009, 'Effect of compassion meditation on neuroendocrine, innate immune and behavioral responses to psychosocial stress', *Psychoneuroendocrinology*, 2009, 34(1), pp. 87–98.

26. Goyal M., Singh S., Sibinga E.M. et al., 2014, 'Meditation programs for psychological stress and wellbeing: A systematic review and meta-analysis', *JAMA Internal Medicine*, 174(3), pp. 357–368.

27. David S., Steve M., Martial V. L. and Arnaud D., 2012, 'Using the daydreaming frequency scale to investigate the relationships between mind-wandering, psychological wellbeing and present-moment awareness', *Frontiers in Psychology*, 3, p. 363.

28. Tang Y. Y., Hölzel B. K. and Posner M. I., 2015, 'The neuroscience of mindfulness meditation', *Nature Reviews Neuroscience*, 16(4), pp. 213–225.

29. Slagter H. A., et al., 2007, 'Mental training affects distribution of limited brain resources', *PLoS Biology*, 5(6), e138.

30. Baas M., Nevicka B. and Ten Velden F. S., 2014, 'Specific mindfulness skills differentially predict creative performance', *Personality and Social Psychology Bulletin*, 40(9), pp. 1092–1106.

31. Lebuda I., Zabelinab D. L. and Karwowski M., 2016, 'Mind full of ideas: A meta-analysis of the mindfulness-creativity link', *Personality and Individual Differences*, 93, pp. 22–26.

32. As a definition of compassion, researchers used 'emotional experience and cognitive anxiety in reaction to others' suffering, and the desire to help the person to feel better'.

33. Rosenberg E. L., Zanesco A. P., King B. G., Aichele S. R., Jacobs T. L., Bridwell D. A., MacLean K. A., Shaver P. R., Ferrer E., Sahdra B. K., Lavy S., Wallace B. A. and Saron C. D., 2015, 'Intensive meditation training influences emotional responses to suffering', *Emotion*, 15(6), pp. 775–790.

Chapter 6 Do what you can!

1. Ricard M., 2011, *The Art of Meditation*, London: Atlantic Books.

2. André C., 2017, *Méditez Avec Nous*, Paris: Odile Jacob.

3. Ibid.

4. Lenoir F., 2018, *Méditer à Cœur Ouvert*, Paris: NiL Éditions.

5. Desai R., Tailor A. and Bhatt T., 2015, 'Effects of yoga on brain waves and structural activation: A review', *Complementary Therapies in Clinical Practice*, 21(2), pp. 112–118.

Chapter 7 It all starts with breathing

1. Chennu S., Annen J., Wannez S., Thibaut A., Chatelle C., Cassol H., Martens G., Schnakers C., Gosseries O., Menon D. and Laureys S., 2017, 'Brain networks predict metabolism, diagnosis and prognosis at the bedside in disorders of consciousness', *Brain*, 140(8), pp. 2120–2132.

2. Lee D. et al., 2018, 'Effects of an online mind–body training program on the default mode network: An EEG functional connectivity study', *Scientific Reports*, 8(1), p. 16935.

3. Annen, J., Laureys, S. et al., 2021, 'Mapping the functional brain state of a world champion freediver in static dry apnea'. Submitted for publication.

4. Piarulli A., Zaccaro A., Laurino M., Menicucci D., De Vito A., Bruschini L., Berrettini S., Bergamasco M., Laureys S. and Gemignani A., 2018, 'Ultra-slow mechanical stimulation of olfactory epithelium modulates consciousness by slowing cerebral rhythms in humans', *Scientific Reports*, 8(1), p. 6581.

5. Raffone A., Marzetti L., Del Gratta C., Perrucci M. G., Romani G. L., Pizzella V., 2019, 'Toward a brain theory of meditation', *Progress in Brain Research*, 244, pp. 207–232.

Chapter 8 Mindfulness here and now

1. Uncapher M. R. and Wagner A. D., 2018, 'Minds and brains of media multitaskers: Current findings and future directions', *Proc. Natl Acad. Sci.*, 115(40), p. 9889–9896.

2. Maex E., 2017, *Mindfulness: Apprivoiser le stress par la pleine conscience*, Paris: De Boeck.

3. Epstein R., 2017, *Attending: Medicine, Mindfulness and Humanity*, New York: Scribner.

Chapter 9 Loving kindness meditation

1. Ogueji, I.A., et al., 2021, 'Coping strategies of individuals in the United Kingdom during the COVID-19 pandemic' *Curr Psychol*, Jan 3: 1–7.

2. Decety J., Bartal I. B., Uzefovsky F. and Knafo-Noam A., 2016, 'Empathy as a driver of prosocial behaviour', *Philosophical Transactions of the Royal Society London B Biological Sciences*, 371 (1686), 20150077.

3. Singer T. and Klimecki O. M., 2014, 'Empathy and compassion', *Current Biology*, 24(18), R875–R878.

4. Russell-Williams J. et al., 2018, 'Mindfulness and meditation: Treating cognitive impairment and reducing stress in dementia', *Reviews in the Neurosciences*, 29(7), pp. 791–804.

Chapter 10 Mindfulness for health workers, athletes, students and inmates

1. Vandenbroeck S., Van Gerven E., De Witte H., Vanhaecht K., Godderis L., 2017, 'Burnout in Belgian physicians and nurses', *Occup Med (Lond)*, 67(7), pp. 546-554.

2. Udemezue O. I., 2017 'Burnout and psychiatric morbidity among doctors in the UK: a systematic literature review of prevalence and associated factors', *BJPsych Bull*, 41(4): pp. 197–204.

3. Sher L., 2011, 'Towards a model of suicidal behavior among physicians', *Revista Brasileira de Psiquiatria*, 33(2), pp. 111–112.

4. Kansoun Z., Boyer L., Hodgkinson M., Villes V., Lançon C. and Fond G., 2019, 'Burnout in French physicians: A systematic review and meta-analysis', *Journal of Affective Disorders*, 246, pp. 132–147.

5. Hafenbrack A. C., Kinias Z. and Barsade S. G., 2014, 'Debiasing the mind through meditation: Mindfulness and the sunk–cost bias', *Psychological Science*, 25(2), pp. 369–376.

6. Birtwell K. et al., 2019, 'An exploration of formal and informal mindfulness practice and associations with wellbeing', *Mindfulness* (NY), 10(1), pp. 89–99.

7. Myriad: www.myriadproject.org.

8. Midal F., 2018, *Foutez-vous La Paix*, Paris: Flammarion.

9. Auty K. M., Cope A. and Liebling A., 2017, 'A systematic review and meta–analysis of yoga and mindfulness meditation in prison', *International Journal of Offender Therapy and Comparative Criminology*, 61(6), pp. 689–710.

10. This penal institution was the subject of a 1997 documentary made by Ayelet Menahemi and Eilona Ariel called *Doing Time, Doing Vipassana*.

11. *See also* Ricard M., 2007, *Happiness: A Guide to Developing Life's Most Important Skill*, London: Atlantic Books.

12. Li C., Zhu Y., Zhang M., Gustafsson H. and Chen T., 2019, 'Mindfulness and athlete burnout: A systematic review and meta-analysis', *International Journal of Enviromental. Research and Public Health*, 16(3), p.ii E449.

13. Djokovic N., 2014, *Serve to Win*, London: Corgi.

14. Solberg E. E., Ingjer F., Holen A., Sundgot-Borgen J., Nilsson S. and Holme I., 2000, 'Stress reactivity to and recovery from a standardised exercise bout: A study of 31 runners practising relaxation techniques', *British Journal of Sports Medicine*, 34(4), pp. 268–72.

15. Bühlmayer L., Birrer D., Röthlin P., Faude O. and Donath L., 2017, 'Effects of mindfulness practice on performance-relevant parameters and performance outcomes in sports: a meta-analytical review', *Sports Medicine*, 47(11), pp. 2309–2321.

16. Kabat-Zinn J., Beall B. and Rippe J., 1985, 'A systematic mental training program based on mindfulness meditation, to optimize performance in collegiate and Olympic rowers', presented at the World Congress in Sport Psychology, Copenhagen, Denmark.

17. Haase L., et al., 2015, 'A pilot study investigating changes in neural processing after mindfulness training in elite athletes', *Frontiers in Behavioral Neuroscience*, 9, article 229.

18. Carraça B., Serpa S., Palmi J. and Rosado A., 2018, 'Enhance sport performance of elite athletes: The mindfulness-based interventions', *Cuadernos de Psicología del Deporte*, 18(2), pp. 79–109.

19. Molcho L., Laureys, S., Intrator N. et al., 2021, 'Real-time EEG monitoring with continuous wearable feedback during marathon', *Proceedings of the 7th Congress of the European College of Sports and Exercise Physicians*. Awaiting publication.

Chapter 11 Tools and tips

1. Ziegler D. A. et al., 2019, 'Closed-loop digital meditation improves sustained attention in young adults', *Nature Human Behaviour*, 3, pp. 746–757.

2. Gál, É. et al., 2021, 'The efficacy of mindfulness meditation apps in enhancing users' well-being and mental health related outcomes: a meta-analysis of randomized controlled trials', *J Affect Disord*. 279, pp. 131–142.

3. Meir-Hasson Y. et al., 2016, 'One-class fMRI-inspired EEG model for self-regulation training', *PLoS One*, 11(5), e0154968.

Bibliographical References

~

Find out more...

Additional scientific references

Alexander R. et al., 2021, 'The neuroscience of positive emotions and affect: Implications for cultivating happiness and wellbeing', *Neurosci. Biobehav. Rev.*, 121, pp. 220–249.

Boly M., Phillips C., Balteau E., Schnakers C., Degueldre C., Moonen G., Luxen A., Peigneux P., Faymonville M. E., Maquet P., Laureys S., 2008, 'Consciousness and cerebral baseline activity fluctuations', *Hum. Brain Mapp.*, 29(7), p. 868–874.

Dahl C. J., Lutz A., Davidson R. J., 2015, 'Reconstructing and deconstructing the self: cognitive mechanisms in meditation practice', *Trends Cogn. Sci.*, 19(9), pp. 515–523.

Demertzi A., Soddu A., Laureys S., 2013, 'Consciousness supporting networks', *Curr. Opin. Neurobiol.*, 23(2), pp. 239–244.

Engen H. G., Bernhardt B. C., Skottnik L., Ricard M., Singer T., 2018, 'Structural changes in socio-affective networks: Multi-modal MRI findings in long–term meditation practitioners', *Neuropsychologia*, 116 (Pt A), pp. 26–33.

Fucci E., Abdoun O., Caclin A., Francis A., Dunne J. D., Ricard M., Davidson, R. J., Lutz A., 2018, 'Differential effects of non-dual and focused attention meditations on the formation of automatic perceptual habits in expert practitioners', *Neuropsychologia*, 119, p. 92–100.

McCall C., Steinbeis N., Ricard M., Singer T., 2014, 'Compassion meditators show less anger, less punishment, and more compensation of victims in response to fairness violations', *Front. Behav. Neurosci.*, 8, p. 424.

Vanhaudenhuyse A., Laureys S., Faymonville M. E., 'Neurophysiology of hypnosis', *Neurophysiol. Clin.*, 2014, 44(4), pp. 343–353.

Websites

Mind Care International Foundation: www.mindcare.foundation

Mind & Life Europe: mindandlife-europe.org

Mind & Life Institute: mindandlife.org

Karuna–Shechen, founded by Matthieu Ricard in 2000, carries out humanitarian projects in India, Nepal and Tibet: karuna-shechen.org

Vipassana Meditation Centre ('Vipassana' means to see things as they really are): dhamma.org

The World Community for Christian Meditation: www.wccm.org

Books

André, C., 2017, *Happiness: 25 Ways to Live Joyfully Through Art*, London: Random House.

André, C., Jollien, A., and Ricard, M., 2018, *In Search of Wisdom: A Monk, A Philosopher, and A Psychiatrist on What Matters Most*, Boulder: Sounds True Inc.

Brach, T., 2003, *Radical Acceptance*, New York: Rider.

Brewer, J., 2021, *Unwinding Anxiety*, New York: Avery.

Brown, A. and Lenoir, F., 2015, *Happiness: A Philosopher's Guide*, London: Melville House.

Djokovic, N., 2013, *Serve to Win*, New York: Zinc Ink.

Dominique, A., 2019, *The Life-Changing Power of Sophrology*, Novato: New World Library.

Epstein, M., 2018, *Advice Not Given: A Guide to Getting Over Yourself*, London: Hay House.

Evans, J., 2017, *The Art of Losing Control : A Guide to Ecstatic Experience*, Edinburgh: Canongate Books.

Farias, M. and Wikholm, C., 2019, *The Buddha Pill: Can Meditation Actually Change You?*, London: Watkins Publishing.

Gallwey, W. T., 1972, *The Inner Game of Tennis: The Classic Guide to the Mental Side of Peak Performance*, New York: Random House.

Goldstein, J., 2013, *Mindfulness: A Practical Guide to Awakening*, Boulder: Sounds True Inc.

Goleman, D. and Davidson, D., 2018, *Altered Traits: Science Reveals How Meditation Changes Your Mind, Brain and Body*, New York: Avery Publishing.

Gunaratana, Bhante H., 2012, *The Four Foundations of Mindfulness in Plain English*, Boston: Wisdom Publications.

Hammer, G., 2020, *GAIN Without Pain: The Happiness Handbook for Health Care Professionals*, Santa Barbara: Same Page LLC.

Harris, D., 2017, *10% happier! How I Tamed the Voice in My Head, Reduced Stress Without Losing My Edge and Found Self-help That Actually Works – A True Story*, London: Yellow Kite.

Harris, R., 2008, *The Happiness Trap: Stop Struggling, Start Living*, London: Robinson Publishing.

Harris S., 2014, *Waking Up: A Guide to Spirituality Without Religion*, New York: Simon & Schuster.

Kabat-Zinn, J., 2004, *Wherever You Go, There You Are: Mindfulness Meditation in Everyday Life*, London: Piatkus.

Korda, J., 2017, *Unsubscribe: Opt Out of Delusion, Tune in to Truth*, Boston: Wisdom Publications.

Kosslyn, S. and Miller, G. W., 2013, *Top Brain, Bottom Brain: Surprising Insights into How You Think*, New York: Simon & Schuster Press.

Lynch, D., 2008, *Catching the Big Fish: Meditation, Consciousness, and Creativity*, New York: TarcherPerigee.

Maex, E. and and Kabat-Zinn J., 2014, *Mindfulness*, Tielt: Lannoo Publishers.

Midal, F., 2021, *The Three-Minute Philosopher: Inspiration for Modern Life*, Philadelphia: Running Press.

Millman, D., 2006, *Way of the peaceful warrior: A Book That Changes Lives*, Novato: HJ Kramer.

Morgan, B., 2016, *The Meditator's Dilemma: An Innovative Approach to Overcoming Obstacles and Revitalizing Your Practice*, Shambhala.

Parks, T., 2011, *Teach Us to Sit Still: A Sceptic's Search for Health and Healing*, London: Vintage.

Ricard, M., 2007, *Happiness: A Guide to Developing Life's Most Important Skill*, Atlantic Books.

Ricard, M. and Singer, W., 2017, *Beyond the Self: Conversations Between Buddhism and Neuroscience*, Cambridge: MIT Press.

Sadhguru, 2021, *Karma: A Yogi's Guide to Crafting Your Destiny*, New York: Harmony.

Siegel, D., 2018, *Aware: The Science and Practice of Presence*, Scribe.

Trubridge, W., 2017, *Oxygen: A Memoir*, New York: HarperCollins Publishers.

Verhaeghen, P., 2017, *Presence: How Mindfulness and Meditation Shape Your Brain, Mind and Life*, Oxford: Oxford University Press.

Wellings, N., 2015, *Why Can't I Meditate? How To Get Your Mindfulness Practice On Track*, London: Piatkus.

Williams, M., Teasdale, J., Segal, Z., Kabat-Zinn, J., 2007, *The Mindful Way Through Depression: Freeing Yourself from Chronic Unhappiness*, New York: Guilford Press.

Williams, M. and Penman, D., 2011, *Mindfulness: A Practical Guide to Finding Peace in a Frantic World*, London: Piatkus.

Zeman, A., 2004, *Consciousness: A User's Guide*, London: Yale University Press.

Selection of scientists working in the area of meditation

Amishi Jha: amishi.com
Bill and Susan Morgan: billandsusan.net
Dan Siegel: drdansiegel.com
David Vago: davidvago.bwh.harvard.edu
Elisha Goldstein: elishagoldstein.com
Judson Brewer: judsonbrewer.com
Jules Evans: philosophyforlife.org
Margaret Cullen: margaretcullen.com
Matthieu Ricard: matthieuricard.org
Richard Davidson: richardjdavidson.com
Ruth Baer: ruthbaer.com
Sam Harris: samharris.org
Sara Lazar: scholar.harvard.edu/sara_lazar
Tania Singer: taniasinger.de
Willoughby Britton: vivo.brown.edu/display/wbritton

Associations

centerhealthyminds.org
ccare.stanford.edu
bodhi-college.org
mindful.org
association-mindfulness.org
headspace.com
calm.com
davidlynchfoundation.org
wakingup.com
imagineclarity.com
petitbambou.com
themindfulnessapp.com

Acknowledgements

Allow me to start off by thanking everyone who taught me how to better experience the power of meditation, to use it in my personal and professional life, and now also to prescribe it in my role of health care provider and neurologist. I'm forever grateful to Matthieu Ricard, my very dear friend, my source of inspiration, my model of embodied ethics, optimism and courage, but also my scientific colleague and incredible guinea pig. I also wish to thank all my friends, colleagues and those practising a contemplative life whom I met at Mind & Life Europe: Amy Cohen Varela (spouse of the late Francisco Varela); Lama Tsoknyi Rinpoche, Diego Hangartner, Martine Batchelor (Tibetan monks); Antoine Lutz, Wolf and Tania Singer, as well as Elena Antonov (neuroscientists); Michel Bitbol and Thomas Metzinger (philosophers); Andreas Roepstorff (anthropologist); Ute Brandes, Charles-Antoine Janssen and Cornelius Pietzner.

Thank you to all other research colleagues and pioneers in meditation for having opened my eyes to a new world. Thank you also to all the people of the superb Yeunten Ling Tibetan Institute in Huy, to Lama Zeupa and to Lea Van Rompay, where I was lucky enough to have been able to do a private retreat upon an invitation extended by Peter Brems (VRT Belgian Public Television).

Thank you to Ilios Kotsou and his wife, Caroline Lesire, for having invited me to their very inspiring conference series, Émergences, in both Brussels and Montreal, which gave me the opportunity to meet fantastic people, most of whom are expert meditators, including Alexandre Jollien and Frédéric Lenoir (philosophers), Christophe André, Edel Maex and Christophe Fauré (psychiatrists), Candice Marro and Ozan Aksoyek (psychotherapists), Nicole Bordeleau, Jean-Marie Lapointe, Rémi Tremblay (authors and conference speakers), Jean-Luc Daub (animal welfare activist), and Maria João Pires and Julien Brocal (pianists).

Thank you as well to all those who contributed interviews for this book, avid meditators Sam Harris (neuroscientist, philosopher and author), David

Lynch (mind-bending filmmaker), Tim Parks (novelist) and Jules Evans (philosopher-author), the decathlete and European champion Thomas Van der Plaetsen, yoga expert Joachim Meire, psychiatrist and mindfulness pioneer and CEO Edel Maex. I am also immensely grateful to all my research colleagues whom I have quoted, and who shared their knowledge and contribution to a better understanding of the effects of meditation on our brain and health.

I would also like to thank, of course, all the participants in our research studies and all the neuroscientists at our GIGA Consciousness Lab at the University of Liège, as well as all the health-workers at the University Hospital at Liège and at our brain centre, the Centre du Cerveau, and the wonderful colleagues from the CERVO Brain Research Centre of Laval University in Canada. Our work on human consciousness still represents an enormous challenge and means we often have to go against the grain, but having such dream-teams to collaborate with makes this work so much more rewarding.

As for our research on meditation, which started with Matthieu Ricard in 2015, it currently continues with other experts, but also with inexperienced meditators, whether it covers the fields of mindfulness, of hypnosis (Dr Audrey Vanhaudenhuyse), of cognitive trance (Dr Olivia Gosseries), or other altered states of consciousness. Our research also continues thanks to our collaborations with colleagues such as Bindu Kutty, professor in neurophysiology at the National Institute of Mental Health and Neurosciences (NIMHANS) in Bangalore, India; with engineer Rajanikant Panda, who is currently finishing his doctoral thesis in our team; with anaesthetist Subramaniam Balachundhar at Harvard University, who works on the effects of yoga on the brain; with my friend the psychologist Ron Kupers, at the University of Copenhagen, and his spouse Dr Laurence Dricot from the Catholic University of Leuven, who studies the effects of heartfulness meditation, comparing it with physical exercise; and last but not least with Matthieu himself and the scientists of Mind & Life Europe, in particular Antoine Lutz, a mindfulness pioneer at the University of Lyon.

Many thanks to all our brilliant undergraduates, PhD students and post-doctoral researchers, all of whom have been a source of inspiration with their humanism, sense of fun and rebellious minds, and the large array of complementary disciplines and diversity of countries and cultures they represent. I am listing them in a more or less chronological order: Dr Caroline Schnakers, neuropsychologist, 'my' first PhD student, who now works in Los Angeles with her husband and colleague, Professor Martin Monti (I am pleased to report that they met each other in the console room of our fMRI); Professor Mélanie Boly, neurologist and Buddhist, my first medical doctor PhD, who also flew off to the US to take up a post at the University of Madison, Wisconsin; among the neuropsychologists, Dr Audrey Vanhaudenhuyse, who leads our research on hypnosis; Dr Olivia Gosseries, who leads our research on cognitive trance; Dr Camille Chatelle; Dr Athena Demertzi in Greece; Charlotte Martial; Lizette Heine (from Maastricht and now in Lyon); Charlène Aubinet, Manon Carrière, Helena Cassol; Alice Barra and Benedetta Cecconi (Italy); Estelle Bonin (France); neuroradiologists Dr Jean Flory Tshibanda, Carol Di Perri (Italy) and Carlo Cavaliere (Italy); physiotherapists Dr Aurore Thibaut (who leads our research on the electrical stimulation of the brain) and Géraldine Martens; the speech therapist Évelyne Melotte; the revalidation medics Nicolas Lejeune (UCL) and Marie-Michèle Briand (Canada); Dr Willemijn Van Erp (Netherlands); Dr Leandro Sanz (Switzerland); biologist Jitka Annen (Netherlands) and Steven Jillings; the computer scientists Stephen Larroque (France) and Federico Raimondo (Argentina); the engineer Rajanikant Panda (our very own meditation expert from India); Sepehr Mortaheb (Iran); Andrea Piarulli and Francesco Riganello (Italy); and finally Cécile Carette, probably the best executive assistant in the known galaxy.

I would like to express my gratefulness to all the visiting fellows, visiting professors on sabbatical, master students, to the whole team and staff at the Sart-Tilman Hospital in Liège (in particular, Professors Marie–Élisabeth Faymonville, Vincent Bonhomme, Roland Hustinx), and to all the colleagues with whom we collaborated in Belgium and abroad. Thanks to them, our research on the contents and states of consciousness, whether in good health or disease, has been a source of enduring fascination for us.

I also want to extend the warmest thanks to all the participants who volunteered, as well as the patients and their families. Our research team has been funded by the Belgian Fund for Scientific Research (FNRS), the

International Fund Generet managed by the King Baudouin Foundation, the Mind Care Foundation, the Belgian Science Policy Office, the Wallonia-Brussels Federation, the Liège Léon-Fredericq Foundation, the University Hospital of Liège, the European Commission, the Human Brain Project, the Marie Curie Networks and the National European Space Agency, the Fondazione Europea di Ricerca Biomedica, the Bial Foundation and the Benoît Foundation, the American foundations James S. McDonnell and Mind Science, and the National Natural Science Foundation of China. Many thanks to all our industrial partners: Toyota, Schmieder Kliniken, g.tec Medical Engineering, Neurosteer, Imagilys and DIM3. And a special thanks to the Fondation Francqui.

This book would not have seen the light of day without Pieter Vanderhaegen, from Borgerhoff & Lamberigts Publishers, who contacted me after having read an interview I gave on meditation and the importance of implementing it in our educational system. Many thanks to Elien Geboers for her editorial help, to Odile Jacob for the French adaptation, and evidently to the exceptional professionals from Bloomsbury Publishing: Matthew Lowing and Zoë Blanc.

Last but not least, I want to thank those who are dearest to me: my wife Vanessa and my fantastic children, in order of appearance, Clara, Hugo, Matias, Louis and Margot, as well as my dear mother.

Do not think of myself and my family's experience as a permanently smooth, calm zen-existence – nothing could be further from the truth and nothing human is strange to us. Remember the main message of this book: we do what we can …

Finally, if you have corrections, constructive criticism, comments, questions or advice, please share it with us and the other readers through my social channels (Facebook, Twitter, LinkedIn, Instagram, YouTube); #drsteven-laureys #nononsensemeditation. Your feedback will undoubtedly make the next edition of this book better! To organise a lecture, please contact me directly or via smartspeakers.ie. Let's stay in touch!

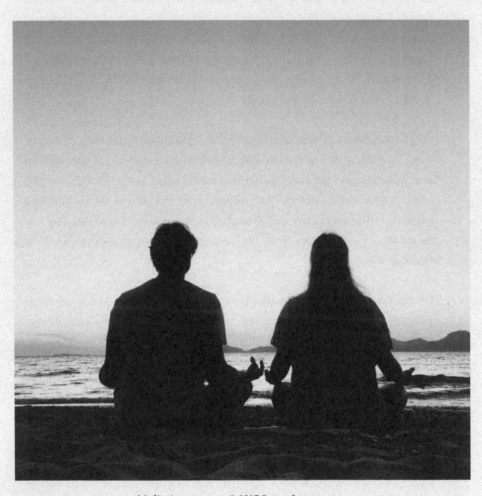

Meditating at sunset. © 2017 Steven Laureys.

'Between stimulus and response there is a space. In that space is our power to choose our response. In our response lies our growth and our freedom.'

VIKTOR FRANKL, NEUROLOGIST AND HOLOCAUST SURVIVOR

You can meditate in a group during a class; you can meditate alone in your room with an audio guide or an app; you can also, as in the picture, meditate as a duo during your honeymoon on a Greek Island, with a timer set on ten minutes... You can do formal meditation sitting on a cushion in the lotus position or you can do it informally, in any spot, when and for as long as you feel like it. You can use any 'lost' moment that comes your way, during a traffic jam, at a red-light signal or at the office, simply step back and think about what you are doing and breathe in consciously. The regular practice of mindfulness helps you to be quicker at spotting those moments when your thoughts are straying from the present moment. It then allows you to refocus on what you are doing in the here and now.

You can offer yourself a brief moment of conscious breathing at any time of the day, when emotions, unpleasant feelings or tensions start building up in your body. This will allow you to face the situations you are presented with in a more controlled manner, instead of unconsciously letting your automatic reflexes take over. Recent scientific studies have shown that these brief but repeated moments of informal meditation and of refocusing our attention are beneficial to our psychic wellbeing and our mental flexibility.

Praise for *The No-Nonsense Meditation Book*

'With "No-Nonsense" Steven Laureys elucidates contemporary varieties of meditation research and applications. The science is captivating in itself, but even more so when rendered in Laureys' candid, lively and empathetic voice. This story of "the brain on meditation" comes alive when it is set in the context of Laureys' personal history and in those of the renowned scientists and scholars and contemplatives who inspire him.'

Amy Cohen Varela, Chair of Mind & Life Europe

'This exciting book – to keep with you at all times – is a true gem, simple, inspiring and packed with solid scientific arguments. Professor Steven Laureys, neuroscientist and clinician, uncovers how the brains of mediators operate. Supported by clinical research and neuroimaging, this is an unmissable guide to find the meditation technique that is right for you.'

Laurence Lucas Skalli MD, psychiatrist and founder of the Medicine and Consciousness Foundation

'I absolutely love this book by Prof. Steven Laureys because it explains meditation from all its angles: both the scientific as well as the practical way, how it impacted not only his but also other people's lives and a handful of tips and tricks. My favorite? "You do what you can". I would recommend this book to everyone interested in the topic, from beginners to experienced meditators.'

Stefanie Broes, PhD, Co-founder, Moonbird

'With a solid scientific background, a sharp sense of observation and a lot of authenticity, this pleasant book helps making mindfulness accessible to everyone, including to sceptics. That makes a lot of sense!'

Benjamin Blasco, Cofounder of Petit BamBou, leading European mindfulness app

'A book that should convince everyone of the benefits of practicing meditation. It contains exercises and ingredients to tame stress and cultivate mental peace in today's challenging world.'

Hugues Cormier MD, psychiatrist, Professor of Mindfulness, University of Montreal

'Full of pragmatic tips, this book will help anyone who is looking to learn how meditation works put it into practice for themselves.'

Judson Brewer MD PhD, Brown University Mindfulness Center,
Author of Unwinding Anxiety and The Craving Mind

'What we refer to as meditation is a longing for experiential realization of the inclusive nature of existence. Thank you, Steven, for sharing of your personal journey and this sincere, significant effort in bringing understanding and acceptance to this timeless, potent practice.'

Sadhguru, Indian yogi and author of
Inner Engineering: A Yogi's Guide to Joy

'A compelling read. A brilliant neurologist venturing into the world of meditation like a true scientist. This book will no doubt bring the beautiful meditation practice into many people's daily lives.'

Bala Subramaniam MD, Harvard Medical School, Boston

'A distinguished specialist in altered states of consciousness, Steven Laureys guides us in a fascinating and clear investigation into meditation. He shows us that our brain is not an organ that determines our lives, but an instrument we can play freely, a potential for fulfillment that it is up to us to cultivate.'

Michel Bitbol MD PhD, French National Centre for Scientific Research

'Steven Laureys is a world-wide expert in neuroscience and studied the human brain for many years with different techniques like EEG and fMRI. It is wonderful that a topic like meditation is explored by a scientist to objectively show the advantages and shortcomings.'

Christoph Guger PhD, Founder & CEO, g.tec medical engineering, Austria

'*The No-Nonsense Meditation Book* by Steven Laureys is an impeccable, incredible and compelling read! This book provides insight on the timeless message of meditation that helps to cultivate – mental lucidity; intellect and cognition; inner wisdom and higher virtues and wholesome behaviors. The scientific evidences and anecdotes are narrated flawlessly. And his natural way of defining meditation – "a simple exercise in awareness" or as "brain fitness" makes the reader feel that anyone can practice meditation and the training helps to attain wisdom and takes you forward. Thank you, Steven, for presenting us with such an insightful book on the science of meditation and its potentials to tap the infinite proficiencies of our brain and mind to attain wisdom.'

Bindu M. Kutty PhD, Professor of Neurophysiology and Head of the Centre for Consciousness Studies, National Institute of Mental Health and Neurosciences, Bangalore, India

'A practical workbook with credible – and accessible – explanations, this book augurs to become an instant classic by effectively connecting personal experience with scientific evidence. The journey of a sceptic is not only more sympathetic, it tends to be more believable. Steven Laureys has done a masterful job with this book. It is a highly welcome contribution to the literature on contemplative science.'

Cornelius Pietzner, Director of Mind & Life Europe

'In this book, Steven Laureys, one of the most celebrated neuroscience researchers in the world, interweaves academic references with practical advice and personal experiences. He offers a unique view of meditation that will propel you towards your meditation cushion.'

Prof Arnaud Delorme PhD, Meditation Researcher, University of California San Diego

'Did you think meditation was fuzzy? Did you think brain-science was boring? Steven Laureys brings together his expertise in meditation and science in an engaging no-nonsense book. A must-read for those who hate floatiness and boredom.'

Edel Maex MD, Zen teacher and psychiatrist, Antwerp University

'Much has been written on the virtues of mindfulness and meditation. Rare are books where personal experience, clinical expertise and scientific rigor fruitfully complement one another to provide a comprehensive assessment of the effects of the multifaceted contemplative practices and of the underlying brain mechanisms. Here is a brilliant example!'

Wolf Singer, Professor of Neuroscience, Max Planck Institute, Germany